THE PROPHET and Her Critics

Other books by these authors:

Leonard Brand
Faith, Reason, and Earth History

Don S. McMahon
Acquired or Inspired? Exploring the Origins of the Adventist Lifestyle

THE PROPHET and Her Critics

A striking new analysis refutes the charges that Ellen G. White "borrowed" the health message

Leonard Brand and Don S. McMahon

Pacific Press® Publishing Association
Nampa, Idaho
Oshawa, Ontario, Canada
www.pacificpress.com

Book design by Dennis Ferree

Library of Congress Cataloging-in-Publication Data

Brand, Leonard, 1941-
The prophet and her critics : a striking new analysis refutes the charges that Ellen G. White "borrowed" the health message/Leonard Brand and Don S. McMahon.
p.cm.
ISBN: 0-8163-2057-8
1. White, Ellen Gould Harmon, 1827-1915. 2. Rea, Walter T. White lie. 3. Butler, Jonathan M. 4. Numbers, Ronald L. Prophetess of health. 5. Health—Religious aspects—Seventh-day Adventists—History of doctrines—19th century. 6. Seventh-day Adventists—Doctrines—History—19th century. I. McMahon, Don S. (Don Stewart), 1938- II. Title.

BX6193.W5B73 2005
286.7'092—dc22 2004057289

Additional copies of this book are available by calling toll free 1-800-765-6955 or by visiting http://www.adventistbookcenter.com.

05 06 07 08 09 • 5 4 3 2 1

Dedication

Leonard Brand dedicates this book to his children,
Dennis and Jenelle, to his nephews and nieces,
and to all others who are seeking to understand
how God communicates with His earthly loved ones.

Don S. McMahon dedicates this book to all those who have
struggled to understand the relevance of Ellen White's writings.

Acknowledgments

We thank our wives for their patience during the many hours we spent at our computers working on this manuscript. We are also grateful for the helpful criticisms of those who read the manuscript, including Richard Nix, Merlin Burt, and the editors at Pacific Press. Please blame us alone for any errors that remain.

Don is also grateful for encouragement from Mandy, Jill, Jamie, Ivan, and the members of his cell group, from Alan Lindsay, Arthur Patrick, and Lester Devine of the White Estate branch office located at Avondale College, and from the many people who providentially offered their expertise at crucial moments.

Table of Contents

CHAPTER 1

Reasons for a New Response

Ellen G. White was one of the founders of the Seventh-day Adventist Church. Her inspired counsels were important to the development of the denomination and its institutions and gave the church confidence in its belief system. Throughout the years, however, several people have written articles or books that claim they've found evidence that her writings do not represent God's revelation to us, but rather were copied from the writings of other persons. They claim to have evidence that discredits her as a spokeswoman for God.

How should we respond to these critics? One response has been to ignore them and hope they go away. Another is to condemn them for questioning her work. But if someone has doubts about the work of a prophet, is it inappropriate for them to study the matter—to research the reliability of the claim of the prophetic gift? What about 1 Thessalonians 5:20, 21: "Do not treat prophecies with contempt. Test everything. Hold on to the good"? God has put Himself and His character on trial before the universe so that His created beings will worship Him out of confidence and trust, not because He has commanded them to. Certainly, then, human prophets are subject to the same type of open investigation of their claims that God has invited regarding Himself.

Of course, in addition to investigating the message of those who claim to speak for God, we must also investigate carefully the claims of those who challenge the prophet's validity. That's what we'll do in the following pages. As we do this, it is of utmost importance that our research be of the highest quality and that we be honestly seeking for truth.

To some readers, it may seem that we are examining criticisms of Ellen White that were answered long ago. People have written responses to the criticisms of her work that we will discuss in this book. However, we find that many people are not familiar with these responses or are not convinced that the responses are adequate. Thus, we offer a new evaluation of several representative critics of Mrs. White's writings.

Christians recognize that in this confusing world we need the guidance of the Holy Spirit if we are to find truth. Someone could charge that our claim to be following the Holy Spirit is really just an excuse to believe what we want to believe. That could happen. However, we believe that we are praying with the right attitude if we pray for the Holy Spirit to give us an open mind that can think clearly, a mind that will deal honestly and fairly with the evidence.

We will not comment on some of the authors' criticisms regarding how the church has handled questions about Mrs. White and those who have criticized her. After all, the church is not infallible, and whether those who have spoken for it have ever made mistakes is another issue. Instead, we'll focus on Mrs. White's work and the question of whether the evidence discredits or supports the claim that she was a divinely inspired prophet who received specific communications from God.

Characteristics of Valid Research

In analyzing the research of Ellen White's critics, we need first to examine the quality of the scholarship represented. Valid research must follow appropriate principles of design. The researchers must have collected the data as carefully and as objectively as humanly possible (although no research is totally objective). The data must be the type that can answer the question that is being asked, and the researcher must use sound logic in interpreting the data.

Sound logic is indispensable. Data never directly dictate the conclusion—the answer to our question. We must use logic to relate data and assumptions or generalizations and then reason to a conclusion. We're well able to do this, especially if we've been trained in the process of logical thought. However, as someone has said, logic can become an organized way of going wrong with confidence. Indeed it can be, if we don't examine our logic carefully. We must recognize the many pitfalls that can trap us into conclusions that the available evidence doesn't support. In fact, we may become discouraged when we realize how much mental effort we must exert to see through the errors of logic in a written work that at first reading seemed well documented and trustworthy.

Here's an example of one common error of logic:

- If a car's spark plug wires are disconnected, the car won't start.
- My car won't start.
- Therefore, someone has disconnected the spark plugs.

The first statement is correct, and so is the observation that the car won't start. What then is the weakness in the conclusion? It could be correct, but we don't know because there are other things that could prevent the car from starting: It could be out of gas, or the distributor could be broken, or any number of other problems. The error is in considering only one possible cause for the observed phenomenon when there are other causes that could be producing it. Other types of errors of logic can also result in faulty interpretation of evidence. We'll encounter several of them in the coming chapters.

Research must be based on a carefully crafted research design—a plan that considers all the hypotheses that are relevant and that identifies what type of data are needed to test these hypotheses and how to gather that data in an objective, unbiased way. Researchers must be very alert to avoid errors in logic as they develop their research design. Yet even the best researcher will not always have a perfect research design; we can't foresee all pitfalls and will recognize some only after we've done the research. In addition, when we've completed and analyzed the initial research, we may realize we need to ask other questions. Then we must improve the design to correct the problem, ask the right questions, repeat the research, and collect the data that can reliably answer those questions.

The first part of this book is primarily an analysis of the research designs used by Ellen White's critics. We won't focus on the spiritual values or religious concepts these authors espouse, but only on the quality of their research. We'll examine their work to see: (1) whether their logic meets an acceptable scholarly standard, avoiding serious logical errors; (2) whether their data support the conclusions they reach; and (3) whether their research design adequately supports their conclusions. In effect, we'll ask if they had submitted their publications as theses in a graduate program, would a team of careful scholars have given them a passing grade?

Then we'll examine new research data that offer a better way to evaluate the source and reliability of Mrs. White's health principles. This new evidence holds promise of yielding solid insights into an area that has been the subject of much speculation: the nature of inspiration. And, finally, we'll look at what she had to say about sexual relationships within marriage.

2 CHAPTER

The White Lie, by Walter Rea

We'll begin our examination of the criticism of Ellen White by looking at research that claims she produced her writings by copying from other human authors. Those who raise this issue conclude that this indicates that God did not inspire the concepts she presented.

Walter Rea conducted this type of research, presenting it in the book *The White Lie.*[1] Rea read books that Ellen White had in her library, compared these with the books she wrote, and compiled a collection of pages on which he found similar ideas or wording. His book contains many examples of these comparisons, facilitating an analysis of his logic. He is to be commended for laying out the evidence so we can analyze his work and determine how he reached his conclusions. I have made one assumption in this analysis: that Rea's book contains the best evidence he found. Certainly, he would have used his best data to support his arguments.

In chapter five, Rea compares the tables of contents of Ellen White's *Patriarchs and Prophets*[2] and *Bible History,* by Alfred Edersheim.[3] The chapter headings certainly follow a similar pattern. Of course, they are both commentaries on the Bible, so it isn't surprising that they follow the same sequence. However, it does appear likely that Edersheim's book may have influenced how Mrs. White organized hers. Later on, we'll discuss whether that is a problem.

Two exhibits display the strongest evidence of Mrs. White's

use of other sources. Each contains several paragraphs in which her book reflects just about word for word what appears in her source. These pages both contain descriptive material, the first describing Zurich, Switzerland, and the surrounding area, and the second, the Waldenses. Another exhibit compares the story of William Miller's life as written by James White, Ellen White's husband, and a section in her book *The Great Controversy*.[4] Ellen White's chapter about William Miller resembles very closely what her husband wrote. Much of the most similar portion is a description of Miller's experience in his own words. If most of Walter Rea's exhibits were of this type, he would indeed have a strong case for extensive copying. But when we look beyond these three exhibits, the nature of his evidence changes quickly.

The remaining 153 pages of exhibits reveal varying degrees of similarity between Mrs. White's books and her presumed sources. In all cases, the similarities are limited to a few lines on a page. In most cases, one must search through several pages to find these few lines of similar material. Outside of these similar phrases or sentences, some exhibits reveal cases in which there are similarities in the general themes presented. It is likely that human sources influenced her organization of the material in some of her books; Rea reveals parallels between the basic concepts in the books, which both parallel the Bible stories.

Included in the appendix to this book is an example of Rea's exhibits. However, this example shows full pages from the source and from Ellen White's book *Prophets and Kings* rather than just the paragraphs that contain parallel material, as Rea's book does. The full pages give a better perspective on what portion of the material is similar.

Four Hypotheses

At one time, Walter Rea believed firmly in the inspiration of Ellen White. But when he discovered the similarities between her work and that of other writers, he rejected divine inspiration as the source of her writings. Do his data lead to this conclusion? Here are four hypotheses of how Mrs. White acquired her ideas:

A1 God dictated all of her writings. They were verbally inspired and original.

A2 God did not dictate her works; she used her own words to express the concepts God gave her. What she wrote was all original; she did not depend on any other sources.

A3 God gave concepts and ideas to her and showed her the equivalent of "motion pictures" of scenes in history to reveal how He was involved in these events. She wrote these in her own words, sometimes utilizing materials from other sources to help her express her ideas better. The God-given, inspired visions were the standard she used in choosing what material to draw from other sources. She also used strictly human writings to fill in the history between the scenes that God showed her. In this case, the words of the prophet were not inspired; rather, God inspired—or educated—the person. (This was Ellen White's own description of how she worked; see the Introduction to *The Great Controversy*.)

A4 God did not inspire her material. She merely copied it from human sources.

The evidence Walter Rea presented seems to falsify hypotheses A1 and A2. It appears that he then jumped to hypothesis A4, which rejects her divine inspiration, without considering that there might be other possibilities. Is that justified? Why did Rea never discuss option A3—Ellen White's own description of how she worked? Was he unaware of her description of her methods?

Rea's conclusion is justified only if his data can distinguish between hypotheses A3 and A4 and can falsify A3, which portrays her as using some material from human sources but selecting that material under the influence of divine inspiration. The evidence we have examined so far is completely compatible with A3. So there's a serious problem in the logic Rea used in *The White Lie*. This major lapse in research design appears to destroy his argument against the divine inspiration of Mrs. White's work. We'll return to this issue shortly.

In addition, Rea and other critics take pains to point out Mrs. White's human qualities and personal mistakes as evidence against considering her an inspired prophet. This issue also calls for an analysis of the logic involved. Do those whom God calls to speak for Him (whether as modern-day prophets or authors of the Bible) suddenly become perfect in their writing and in their lives? Or are they still human and in need of continuing growth? (Ask Bathsheba about that!)

Instead of jumping from one extreme ("inspired, and thus perfect in all respects") to the other ("not perfect, thus not inspired"), we need to compare some of the possible hypotheses spanning the distance between. In this case, we list a representative sampling of these hypotheses:

B1 Prophets live perfect lives. Everything they write is inspired, even their private communications to friends. Prophets never have incorrect ideas, even in their private lives.

B2 Prophets are human, with imperfect private lives. In addition to their inspired writings, prophets also write personal things that are not inspired. The Holy Spirit supervises the selection and preservation of inspired material. God educates prophets gradually as He communicates more information to them. As this occurs, the added information influences the prophets' private lives as well.

B3 Prophets who live imperfect lives and fail to follow the advice God supposedly communicated to them is evidence that their prophetic claim is false. And when a so-called prophet's personal correspondence contains faulty beliefs, that also indicates that the prophet's "inspiration" is merely human.

When Walter Rea found that Mrs. White made mistakes in her private life, he jumped to hypothesis B3, rejecting her prophetic role without considering that there might be other valid explanations. The fact that neither Mrs. White's life nor her response to God's instructions was faultless doesn't mean that we must jump to conclusion B3. We need to consider hypothesis B2 and examine the evidence in light of this possibility. Refuting hypothesis B1 does not lead to hypothesis B3 unless the evidence also eliminates hypothesis B2.

In later chapters of his book, Walter Rea attempts to answer objections to his conclusions. In chapter 12 he states, "Perhaps one of the hardest charges to meet and refute is that Ellen wrote what she had first seen in vision, and that she used the words, thoughts, and arrangement of others only because they said what she wanted to say and did not have the ability to say."[5] Rea admits that this argument "in fact contradicts most of the arguments that have gone before." That is, this objection refutes his arguments against her inspiration.

However, Rea feels that he answers this objection when he shows that in her books, Ellen White used some material written by her husband, James. The problem here is that Walter Rea has committed another very basic error in his logic. He thinks that he has answered the question "Did Ellen White have divine guidance in selection of material to use in her books?" In fact, however, the evidence he presented answers a different question: "Did James White ever write anything of sufficient quality and accuracy that Ellen could use it in her books?" In other words, Walter Rea utterly fails to answer the objection that he admitted "contradicts most of the arguments that have gone before" in his book.

Another Serious Objection

In chapter 13, Rea attempts to deal with another serious objection to his conclusions. This objection is that the quality of Ellen White's writing and the power of its spiritual message confirm the role of the Holy Spirit in inspiring this material. Rea quotes two advocates of this position: " 'Any honest critic must come away from a reading of *Great Controversy* impressed with the power of its message.' "[6] " 'We think that the unprejudiced reader of *The Great Controversy* . . . *will have no difficulty in concluding that the book gives evidence of a grand design that was not copied from human writings.* . . . There is a pulsing life in that book that cannot be found in secular or church histories. . . . We believe the life that pulses in that book is God breathed—inspired of God. That there should be the human touch of human hands before this miracle of life actually speaks to men, detracts nought from the miracle' "[7] (emphasis supplied by Rea).

Rea acknowledges that "this plank in the platform is one of the most difficult to come to grips with." Then, in the rest of the chapter, he discusses such topics as the relationship between the authority of the Bible and the authority of Ellen White in the minds of the church and its leaders, the question of whether the "pushing and goading" of the Adventist leaders who believe in Ellen White has produced a people superior in spiritual matters, and his claim that the church must eliminate the authority of Ellen White if they're to let the biblical Christ into the church. (The latter is a false claim; Christ's role as our Savior and the source of righteousness comprises a prominent theme in Mrs. White's writings.) None of these topics provides any evidence that could answer this "plank in the platform" that Rea acknowledges is one of the strongest arguments against his claims.

One could argue, I believe, that some people use Ellen White's writings to push the biblical Christ out of the way. But to do so, they must selectively quote them out of context, and that is very different from the claim that the thoughtful reader can find no evidence of a divine influence in her writings. Rea "proves" his point about the difficulty the apparent authenticity of the inspiration of Mrs. White's books poses to his argument by rambling through the rest of the chapter without ever coming to grips with it.

Did Rea think he had answered this "difficult plank"? I don't know. One thing is clear, however: Rea's research design and his logic contain errors that are fatal to his argument. His evidence is consistent with hypothesis A3 above—Mrs. White's own description of the relationship between inspiration and her use of other "sources." In fact, the evidence that Rea uses could never disprove hypothesis A3.

The evidence in many of the exhibits in Rea's book clearly indicates that Mrs. White had read the other religious books represented there. Even though only a small part of her material is actually close to being a copy, the general expressions and organization of her material often reflect those other books. It is difficult to deny that part of her wording and at least some of her ideas mirror them. However, if, as she herself said, she used these other sources merely to help her express her divinely inspired thoughts, her use of other books doesn't reduce the miracle of inspiration or the trustworthiness of her message.

Rea also claims that Ellen White's use of the wording of other authors was unethical. Others who have examined this issue have concluded that in the time in which she worked, her methods were considered appropriate. This is a different issue from our theme of analysis of the research methods of her critics, and we will not consider the ethical issue further. Instead, I'll recommend that you evaluate this from the analyses that have been published.[8]

This analysis of Rea's research design does not prove that Ellen White was a true prophet. It does show, however, that Rea has not provided evidence that indicates Mrs. White was *not* a true prophet. He has not given us reason to doubt that God inspired her or that she wrote trustworthy material. Walter Rea's work does not approach the standard of logical consistency that careful scholars would expect in a work that is to be taken seriously.

What kind of evidence would one need to determine with finality whether hypothesis A3 or hypothesis A4 fits her case? The final objection that Rea tries to answer in his chapter 13 is a beginning. Walter Rea did not find an answer to this assertion that the quality of Mrs. White's writing and the power of its spiritual message indicate more than a human source. It stands as a challenge to his conclusions. No one has yet refuted it.

Deuteronomy 18:22 says, "If what a prophet proclaims in the name of the Lord does not take place or come true, that is a message that the Lord has not spoken." The ultimate test of Ellen White's inspiration is in the truth of her words. Do her predictions come true?

Her most dramatic predictions deal with events at the end of the world, and we will only know how true these are when that time comes. It is interesting to watch trends in world conditions and see how they parallel what she had to say, but we have not come to the end yet. We'll consider this issue further in chapter three.

Other questions we might ask: Has her leadership resulted in a successful religious organization? Did her leadership in developing the Seventh-day Adventist educational system result in a thriving, effective system, and have her principles of education stood the test of time? Mrs. White gave her church a system of healthful living a century before science was sufficiently advanced to test many of the health principles she promoted. How does modern medicine evaluate these principles? (We'll look more closely at this issue in chapters four and five.)

Did her direct leadership in the beginning of our various medical institutions and schools result in successful institutions that were a benefit to the work of the Seventh-day Adventist Church?

Questions like these have the potential to determine whether hypothesis A3 or hypothesis A4 fits the case—to determine, in other words, whether Ellen White was divinely inspired. For the reasons given above, simply showing that she borrowed the wording of other writers can never answer that question.

Another View: The White Truth

John J. Robertson wrote his book *The White Truth* before Walter Rea's *The White Lie* was published, although the title chosen by the publisher makes it appear that it was a response to *The White Lie.* The two books do address some of the same issues from very different viewpoints, so we will evaluate Robertson's approach. He maintains that Ellen White did not lie or otherwise mislead us, that she was not a plagiarist, and that the evidence supports her standing as a true prophet of God. Does he use a research design that provides the evidence to support his conclusions reliably? I'll begin by summarizing the principal points of the book and then we'll look at his research design.

Robertson presents the description Ellen White gave in the introduction of *The Great Controversy* as to how she used sources. As we noted earlier, she explains that she chose material consistent with what she had seen in vision and quoted or briefly summarized it. Then Robertson addresses the charge of plagiarism. He cites law experts who conclude that examination of her writings in light of the publishing practices and copyright law of the 1800s shows that there is no basis for a charge of plagiarism. In fact, no publisher or author ever brought this charge against her.

Robertson also presents evidence that Ellen White and/or her publisher were publishing recommendations for Adventists to read several of the books from which she was "borrowing." If she or her publisher were trying to hide her "borrowing," it doesn't seem likely that they would be advertising her very sources to her readers.

In the third and fifth chapters of his book, Robertson compares different views of revelation and inspiration and their application to Mrs. White's work. Did God really communicate concepts to her? Do her writings present reliable and trustworthy information? Or, as some critics suggest, were the ideas she presented her subjective ideas and not God-given truth and thus suitable only for pastoral counseling and not for determining truth?

Regarding that question, Mrs. White rejected any soft, middle ground. She stated clearly that her writings are either "of the Spirit of God, or of the devil."[9] If her ideas are not from God, and thus not trustworthy, why would we think that we should use them in pastoral counseling? Either she was what she claimed to be, or she and all her work were a fraud. She recommended that we test her writings against Bible truth and reject them if they don't meet the test.

Robertson appeals to the results of her work in guiding the Seventh-day Adventist Church to unity in belief and to success in its spiritual venture. He also cites the example of one of the visions she received and the circumstances surrounding its presentation that seem to require a supernatural explanation.

The vision pictured a committee meeting that took place in Battle Creek, Michigan. Mrs. White received the vision in Salamanca, New York, several months prior to the meeting of the committee. She was not told in the vision when the meeting was to occur; she thought it had already occurred. Several times she attempted to describe the contents of the vision in public, but she was prevented from remembering it until the day of the meeting. At the time when the meeting concluded, at night, she was awakened and instructed to present at the church meeting later that morning the vision that she had seen several months before. She did so, and the persons who had attended the committee meeting recognized their part in it and accepted the counsel she gave.

Here's another significant question that people have debated for years: What was Ellen White's role, compared to that of the Bible, in determining doctrinal truth? Since she played an important part in the original establishment of Adventist beliefs, does the church place her above the Bible?

Robertson summarized the history of this process, pointing out that the leaders of the church in its early years developed the beliefs of the church through extensive Bible study. Mrs. White did not receive visions on any topic until after this Bible study, and then her role was to resolve disputes or to lend support to the positions that the leaders had staked out. She drew attention to Bible statements that supported or contradicted the points that people were raising. She herself said that her primary mission was to bring her readers back to the Bible as the authority for doctrines. She insisted that people always maintain Scripture as the standard and that they must test her work against Scripture rather than Scripture by her work. It doesn't seem likely that in those early years of what became the Seventh-day Adventist movement, a frail young woman could have easily swayed the strong-willed church founders, unless they saw good evidence of God's leading in her work.

Ultimately, Robertson concluded that Mrs. White used the writings of others in producing her own works, but that "in her writings is a power and originality which the church recognizes as the prophetic voice." He cites a lawyer who sought to find evidence of plagiarism in Mrs. White's writings but concluded that there was no such evidence. Instead, this lawyer stated, "She moved me. And I think her writings should move anyone, unless he is permanently biased and unswayable."

Analysis of Robertson

What can we conclude about Robertson's evaluation of Ellen White and her writings? Did he make better use of logic and evidence than Walter Rea did?

Both authors had personal opinions about Mrs. White and her works, and each presented a case in favor of his opinion. But we cannot consider either book a research document that carefully compares her work against the evidence. Robertson gives us an alternate interpretation of the work of Mrs. White and its relationship to the Bible and to truth. He supports this interpretation with some evidence, such as the Salamanca vision described above, and other evidence of a similar type. Most of this evidence requires a willingness to believe that she was objective in her descriptions of the events in her life. Both books are apologetic efforts to present a particular view of her life and work, rather than scholarly attempts to test the hypothesis of divine inspiration.

We must commend Robertson for an analysis that, compared to Rea's, is more responsible. Robertson included Mrs. White's own description of how she received her information from God and how reading the works of other authors aided her writing. I have to ask myself, why didn't Rea do that? It hardly seems possible that he was unaware of her *Great Controversy* statements about how she used other sources. If he had considered those statements, they would have required some changes in his interpretation of the evidence.

Fred Veltman's Study of *The Desire of Ages*

Fred Veltman did a study of Ellen White's use of sources that was much more scholarly and objective than Walter Rea's.[10] Veltman made extensive comparisons between fifteen randomly chosen chapters in Mrs. White's book *The Desire of Ages* and the sources she consulted while writing the book.

Mrs. White read widely in books on the life of Christ, and Veltman concludes that she clearly did utilize a number of these sources. He found that 31.4 percent of the sentences in *The Desire of Ages* show some similarity to nonbiblical sources, 7.2 percent are at least partly derived from the Bible, and 61.4 percent showed no similarity in wording to any of her sources.

Veltman rated the degree of similarity of a sentence to some nonbiblical source on a scale of zero (original—no source found) to seven (copied verbatim from some source). The sentences that showed some similarity to a source averaged 3.33 on the 0 to 7 scale. Veltman characterized that average as a loose paraphrase. However, the content of *The Desire of Ages*—the concepts expressed and the organization of thoughts—shows more similarity to her source books than the percentages given would seem to indicate.

Ellen White made considerable use of her source books, even though she did not often closely follow their specific wording. She didn't blindly copy the thoughts in those sources, but made selective and creative use of her own writings and the writings of others to produce what Veltman described as a "customized" composition that expressed *her* belief system. Her unique fingerprint is most evident in the devotional, moral, or Christian appeals that are abundant in *The Desire of Ages*. Her writing also contrasts with her sources in her treatment of eternal realities, such as heaven, and the work of God, the angels, and the devil. Her writing on these topics reads as a factual record, while that of the other life-of-Christ books reads more as suppositions or probabilities. Her writing style is also more readable and understandable than that of her sources.

Veltman recognized that the data he used cannot tell us whether or not Mrs. White received the concepts in *The Desire of Ages* in vision and used other sources only to help her express those divinely given thoughts. In other words, study of her source books can help us understand her editorial methods—how she achieved the wording in her books. It cannot test between hypotheses A3 and A4 given earlier in this chapter.

How, then, do we explain Ellen White's work? Does it consist of merely human-produced documents, or must we understand it to have involved an extrahuman source of information? Robertson's book is helpful, but it should be possible to conduct more carefully designed research that can eliminate one of these two interpretations. I'll present one such study in the latter portion of this book.

---

1. Walter T. Rea, *The White Lie* (Turlock, Calif.: M & R Publications, 1982).

2. Ellen G. White, *Patriarchs and Prophets* (Nampa, Idaho: Pacific Press®, 1958).

3. Alfred Edersheim, *Bible History: Old Testament*. Vols. 1–4 (Grand Rapids, Mich.: Eerdmans, 1949 [reprint]).

4. Ellen G. White, *The Great Controversy* (Nampa, Idaho: Pacific Press®, 1950).

5. Rea, 222 (page 19 of this book).

6. D. R. McAdams, "Ellen G. White and the Protestant Historians" (Unpublished manuscript, Andrews University, 1974), 232, 233.

7. F. D. Nichol, *Ellen G. White and Her Critics* (Hagerstown, Md.: Review and Herald, 1951), 463.

8. See John J. Robertson, *The White Truth* (Nampa, Idaho: Pacific Press®, 1981), 25–40; see also attorney Vincent L. Ramik's report: <http://www.whiteestate.org/issues/ramik.html>.

9. Ellen G. White, *Testimonies for the Church* (Nampa, Idaho: Pacific Press®, 1948), 5:671.

10. See the summary of Fred Veltman's study under "Summary and Conclusions" in "Life of Christ Research Project" at <http://www.adventistarchives.org/doc-info.asp?DocID=1188>.

3
CHAPTER

A Failed Prophecy?

In 1979, Jonathan Butler made the claim that Ellen White derived her understanding of end-time events from conditions in her own day based on her assumption that she was living in the time of the end.[1] Butler gathered information on the political and religious conditions current in her lifetime and found that many matched what she predicted for the end time. For instance, people were calling for Sunday laws to protect law and order in this country, and this matched her description of end-time events. In addition, spiritualism was on the increase, and she declared that spiritualism would play an important role in end-time events.

Butler concluded, "When Mrs. White heralded the end of the world, she spoke of the end of *her* world" (emphasis in the original)—the end of the Protestant America she knew. However, Butler said, those trends did not continue but declined in prominence, and Ellen White's nineteenth-century Protestant American world did not end with the Second Coming. Butler then continued with a strong claim: "What Seventh-day Adventists must fully acknowledge here . . . is the element of *prophetic disconfirmation*" (emphasis in the original). In other words, Ellen White's prophecy failed.

Butler's arguments differ from Walter Rea's in a way that significantly affects how we approach evaluating them. Butler focuses on Ellen White's statements about what she believed will happen just before the Second Coming, whenever that will be. Thus, no one can make a complete assessment of his conclusions until after the end-time events occur; only then will we be able to see who is correct, White or Butler.

However, we can deal with some of the issues now. For example, Butler claimed that if we followed proper interpretation of Scripture, we would have recognized communism, not the papacy, as one of the relevant beasts of Revelation 13. After all, the papacy had little evident power at the time Butler wrote his article, and communism was a serious problem for Christianity. I remember reading Butler's article in 1979 and thinking, *We'll wait and see who is the false prophet, White or Butler.*

Events since 1979 have shown Butler to be wrong in this instance. We all know what has happened to communism since then. I'm not denying that in the 1970s, communism was a serious problem for Christianity. But if we had accepted and broadcast the interpretation that it was one of the beasts that Revelation pictures as at work just before the Second Coming, we would have been left looking foolish. Of course, we can't yet rule out the possibility that communism might regain its power, but at the present time the waning power of communism and the growing prestige of the pope of Rome don't bode well for Butler's interpretation.

Ellen White's discussion of Revelation 13 speaks of events at a specific time in history: the end of time, just before the Second Coming. We are not in that time yet. And certainly, we didn't need to connect communism with the beast of Revelation 13 to see that communism was destructive to Christianity. In reality, Butler did precisely what he accused White of doing. He read the newspapers of his day and interpreted Revelation 13 in light of current events rather than allowing Revelation 13 to provide the basis for its own interpretation.

Someone may claim that what I've said here is incorrect because I am misinterpreting what Butler was saying. He was evaluating Ellen White's writings not as predictions of the future, but merely as commentary on events in her day. I recognize this, but the question is whether he used a valid research design to reach his conclusion.

Fact or Interpretation?

Scientists recognize the importance of distinguishing between data and personal interpretations of data. They must never present their personal interpretations or hypotheses as if they were data, or facts. Certainly, the type of historical analysis seen in Butler's discussion of Ellen White's writings requires this same distinction. However, the very core of Butler's article is a presentation of a hypothesis as if it were fact. His hypothesis is that Ellen White did not intend to predict future events, but that her purpose was to comment on events and trends of her own time. "Ellen White made primarily contemporary comment and protest. Prophesying for Mrs. White was not crystal-ball gazing into a remote future." "To be sure, Mrs. White's eschatology included the *future* as well as the *present tense*, but it was the *near future*"[2] (emphasis in original). Here we see Butler's hypothesis—that prophets, including Ellen White, commented on their own time and did not predict the distant future. But Butler presented his hypothesis as if it were fact. He surely knew that the Seventh-day Adventist Church thinks otherwise, but he provided us no evidence that his hypothesis is correct and the more traditional Adventist alternative is wrong.

Apparently, he thought he did provide such evidence: namely, the evidence that some of the conditions to be expected in the end time were prominent in Ellen White's day, and she recognized that they were prominent. Again, however, we must beware of simple either/or, black-or-white reasoning. Butler claims that Ellen White's predictions have been "disconfirmed" because the Sunday legislation movement declined after her day, the end-time persecution did not begin, and America has not repudiated its constitutional government. Whether her statements have been disconfirmed depends entirely on whether she was predicting a distant event just before the Second Coming or whether she was commenting on contemporary events, as Butler claims.

Butler's analysis of Ellen White's writings is a prime example of oversimplifying an issue by reducing it down to the two positions at its extremes and failing to consider other, intermediate hypotheses. This is the same mistake that Walter Rea made in interpreting Ellen White's "borrowing" (see hypotheses A1 and A4 in the previous chapter). One of the intermediate interpretations that Butler should have considered is that Sunday laws, spiritualism, etc., were prominent in Ellen White's day and will again be important just before the Second Coming, but might go into a temporary decline in the intervening years.

Actually, Butler mentioned this possibility but quickly dismissed it—not by presenting any evidence to support his dismissal, but with his hypothesis that apocalypticism must focus on the present.[3] He feared that doing otherwise might weaken the sense of imminency regarding the end of time. But perhaps apocalypticism is not as shallow as that. Perhaps apocalyptic writings are intended to prepare us for a specific event whenever that event will occur, whether soon or much later. The apostle Paul understood it this way, and he felt constrained to tell his parishioners that the Lord will not come back right away; that he will not return until certain events have happened (see 2 Thessalonians 2:1–12).

In the midst of a discussion of end-time events and persecution, Ellen White stated, "To human wisdom all this now seems impossible; but as the restraining Spirit of God shall be withdrawn from men . . . there will be strange developments."[4] This statement seems to indicate clearly that she did not see all the conditions of her day leading naturally to the end-time events. She was predicting a future that did not seem possible in her day.

It is quite possible that Ellen White believed the Second Coming would occur in her generation, but this does not mean that events then current were the source of her understanding of last-day events. If we are going to use sound reasoning, we will need to consider the possibility that she received her understanding by revelation and that the resemblance of the revealed data to some current events, while important to her, was not the source of her prophetic information. My main point here is that Butler is rejecting hypotheses that differ from his own not because of evidence, but simply because he prefers his interpretation. In the process, he ignores evidence in Ellen White's writings that contradicts his claim that she saw conditions in her day as leading naturally to the end time.

When the Second Coming arrives, we will know for sure whether Ellen White was merely commenting on conditions in her day or whether she was preparing us for an event that in her day was in the distant future. In the meantime, it is evident that Butler's confident conclusion of *prophetic disconfirmation* was premature, and that perhaps we would be wise to study carefully what she has said.

---

1. See Jonathan Butler, "The World of E. G. White and the End of the World," *Spectrum*, 10(2):2–13.
2. Ibid., 3, 10, respectively.
3. Ibid., 11.
4. White, *The Great Controversy*, 608.

CHAPTER 4

Prophetess of Health, by Ronald Numbers

The book *Prophetess of Health*, by Dr. Ronald Numbers,[1] provides an illuminating account of the developing health-reform movement of the 1800s. In this book, Numbers also gives his evaluation of Ellen G. White's relationship to this movement. He suggests that she received the health-reform principles that she advocated from this movement rather than, as she claimed, from God-given visions. To evaluate this charge, we must acquaint ourselves with the health practices of the time in which she lived.*

As the nineteenth century dawned, Americans lived a very unhealthful lifestyle, with little concept of hygiene and an even worse diet. They bathed little and ate large amounts of meat and fat and few fruits and vegetables. The practice of medicine at that time was of little help in dealing with the resulting health problems. The existence of germs was not demonstrated until Pasteur did so in the mid-nineteenth century. The experience of Dr. Ignaz Semmelweis illustrates what resulted from this ignorance of the role of germs in causing disease.[2]

Semmelweis was in charge of the maternity ward in a large and famous teaching hospital in Vienna in the 1840s. At that time, the death rate in maternity wards was appallingly high: One out of six patients died. The observant Dr. Semmelweis began to notice revealing patterns. Each morning he and the medical students performed autopsies on the women who had died during the

*Except where I've given another reference, I've based my summary of this history on *Prophetess of Health*.

previous twenty-four hours, and then, without washing their hands (standard medical procedure at the time), they examined some of the remaining patients. He noticed that the women who had been examined were more likely to die than those who had not been examined.

Semmelweis wondered if the medical staff was carrying something from the dead patients to the live ones. He brought in some washbasins and required all the medical staff to wash their hands after examining the dead. There was much complaining about this bothersome procedure, but within three months the death rate dropped by fourteenfold! Then one day they examined twelve women, and although they had washed their hands between the autopsies and the examinations, eleven of these women became sick and died. Semmelweis again wondered if they might have carried something from one living mother to the others, so he began requiring the physicians and students in his ward to wash after every patient. The death rate went lower still.

Instead of receiving appreciation for his success, however, Semmelweis's colleagues and students ridiculed him, and eventually he was dismissed from his job. After his departure, the washbasins were thrown out, and the death rate went back up to its former level.

Semmelweis was unable to get a job in any other Vienna hospital, so he went to Budapest, where he was put in charge of the maternity ward in a local hospital. He repeated his handwashing experiment, with the same success in lowering death rates. He carefully documented this work in a book, but the medical field was not ready for all of his bothersome washings, and he again was ridiculed and removed from his position at the hospital. He died in a mental institution with the memory of all the unnecessary deaths of those mothers weighing heavily on his mind. Doctors now recognize that routine washing before, between, and after patients is the most important infection-control procedure.

During the early and middle nineteenth century, doctors commonly used bleeding (bloodletting) to treat various health problems. We now recognize that this was a dangerous practice. They also blistered and purged—other questionable practices. The medicines in vogue then, such as the abundantly available patent medicines, did very little good. I have a reprint of the 1897 Sears and Roebuck catalog; even at that late date it was advertising a plethora of drugs that promise to cure virtually everything. Many of the drugs used during that century in the attempt to treat diseases were positively harmful—among them the poisons strychnine and arsenic. A medical historian has said that the practice of medicine crossed an important milestone in about the year 1915. After that date going to a doctor increased rather than decreased a sick person's probability of survival and recovery. Whether or not that date is correct, it seems true that nineteenth-century medicine was of questionable value.

American Health Reformers

It was against this background that a popular health-reform movement began. In America, the first prominent reformer was Sylvester Graham, a Presbyterian minister. After suffering from repeated illnesses, he improved his health by changing his diet and lifestyle. Then, in the 1830s, he began lecturing on health reform. He itinerated widely in eastern American cities and gained a significant following, although his strange reforms also raised a public outcry. He published his message in 1839 as *Lectures on the Science of Human Life*.

Graham prescribed a vegetarian diet, pure water as the only suitable drink; meals no more frequently than every six hours; rest; frequent physical exercise; cleanliness; and the avoidance of tight, restrictive clothing, of all stimulating and "unnatural" foods, and of most dairy products. He advised sleeping in a well-ventilated room at regular hours and avoiding "marital excess" (which he usually defined as having sexual intercourse more than once a month). He warned men that if they shaved their beards, they would reduce their manly powers and shorten life. And he dismissed all medications as evil and not to be used.

A series of other health reformers followed Graham. All of them rejected the standard medical principles of that time and advocated their own versions of healthful living. In the late 1830s, William A. Alcott, a physician trained at Yale University, turned to the methods of the health reformers to regain his own health and then began advocating health reform. Other reformers included Horace Mann, Dio (Diocletian) Lewis, and Larkin B. Coles—a Millerite preacher who was also trained as a physician. Coles wrote two books: *Philosophy of Health: Natural Principles of Health and Cure* and *The Beauties and Deformities of Tobacco-Using.*

The health reformers of that time offered various approaches to treating illnesses and injuries. A majority of them adopted hydropathy—water treatments—and they set up a number of water-cure treatment centers. Of special interest to us is the water cure operated by the reformer Russell T. Trall. He combined this therapy with other health reforms into a system of "hygienic medication," and he edited the *Water Cure Journal,* which another reformer, Joel Shew, had started. Trall also established a hydropathic school, called the New York Hygeio-Therapeutic College. One of the subjects taught there was phrenology, which was also of considerable interest to other health reformers of the time. Phrenology was the study of the skull; practitioners believed they could identify the characteristics of a person's brain and character by examining the shape of that person's skull.

After the American civil war there was less interest in water cures, but a few survived—notably Dr. James C. Jackson's Our Home on the Hillside, in Dansville, New York. Jackson published a health paper called *Laws of Life* (initially called the *Letter Box*). He based his comprehensive health model on ten natural remedies: air; food; water; sunlight; dress; exercise; sleep; rest; and social, mental, and moral influence.

Ellen White also advocated health reform. She did so, she said, as the result of visions she received from God laying out the principles of healthful living that became an important part of the lifestyle of most Seventh-day Adventists. It is evident, however, that she didn't originate health reform. These other health reformers were actively presenting their message well before she began presenting hers.

In *Prophetess of Health,* Ron Numbers attempted to address the question of the influence of these other health reformers on what Mrs. White wrote. Her personal library contained a number of the publications of the health reformers I've mentioned, and she is known to have read these publications. Some of her written material on health contains passages that closely resemble statements made in these other health-reform publications. They seem to reflect her close acquaintance with these writings. Was Mrs. White, then, dependent on these sources for the health principles she promoted, or did God truly reveal them to her as she claimed?

Prophetess of Health clearly implies that Mrs. White's health-reform principles were not God-given, but that she copied them from other health reformers of her day. Was Numbers's approach objective? Does his conclusion stand up to careful scrutiny? Before we can answer that, we'll take a closer look at Mrs. White's work.*

Ellen White had her first health vision in 1848; it warned primarily against the use of tobacco (and maybe tea and coffee also). Her second health vision, in 1854, counseled against the eating of rich foods. Her major health vision came in June 1863; it presented the basic health concepts published in *Spiritual Gifts* in 1864, which initiated a strong focus on healthful living among Seventh-day Adventists.

How extensively were she and her friends acquainted with the work of other health reformers before that? Beginning in the early 1840s, several of Mrs. White's close associates were reading and adopting some of the health-reform principles. For example, Joseph Bates began following Graham's health principles in 1843, and John Loughborough began eating Graham bread and reading the *Water Cure Journal* in 1848. Numbers states that these men "undoubtedly spoke to the Whites of their experiences in health

*Also summarized from Numbers's book.

reform." However, he doesn't present any evidence to support that statement. Apparently, then, we don't know for sure how aware the Whites were of the principles the health-reform movement was promoting at that time.

In January 1863, Jackson published an article on the treatment of diphtheria, which Mrs. White read. She used the treatments in this article to nurse her two sons through apparent attacks of diphtheria. The Whites were very grateful, and James White reprinted Jackson's article in the Seventh-day Adventist Church paper, the *Review and Herald.* Then in February and May of 1863, James White published more health-reform articles in the *Review and Herald.* These articles dealt with the importance of air, water, and light, which James called "God's great remedies." They also advocated dressing healthfully; a meatless, low-fat diet; and restricting oneself to two meals a day. Numbers points to these articles as evidence that by the time of Ellen White's most significant health-reform vision in June 1863, "Seventh-day Adventists were already in possession of the main outlines of the health reform message."[3]

Answering the Charge

After Ellen White began speaking on the topic of health reform, some who heard her asked if she had read the publications of the various health reformers. She answered "that she had not, and would not until she had fully written out her views, 'lest it should be said that I had received my light upon the subject of health from physicians, and not from the Lord.' "[4] Numbers claims that this statement was false, because Mrs. White had read Jackson's article on diphtheria. However, since that article was focused on diphtheria and did not deal with the broad topic of health reform, perhaps Numbers was being too hard on her. In 1864, she wrote out her health-reform principles and published them in *Spiritual Gifts.*

Late in 1863, before *Spiritual Gifts* was published, James White saw advertisements for some of Jackson's publications, and he ordered them. He was busy and did not open the packages when they arrived. Ellen White stated, "As I determined not to read them until I had written out my views, the books remained in their wrappers." After publishing *Spiritual Gifts,* the Whites purchased and read the books and journals of a number of other health reformers. They also, in late autumn 1864, spent three weeks at Jackson's water cure, Our Home on the Hillside. After this Ellen became an advocate of hydropathic treatments; she gave such treatments to neighbors in Battle Creek.

Later, Ellen White published a series of pamphlets called *How to Live*. Among them were a health essay that she wrote and selections by a number of the prominent health reformers of the time. She stated that she did not publish the writings of other reformers to indicate the sources of her health concepts. She explained, "I . . . searched the various works on Hygiene and was surprised to find them so nearly in harmony with what the Lord had revealed to me. And to show this harmony . . . I determined to publish *How to Live,* in which I largely extracted from the works referred to."

Thus it is evident, and acknowledged by Ellen White herself, that after she put her health vision of 1863 down on paper, she became well acquainted with the health writings of others and even republished some of their material. The Whites also visited Our Home on the Hillside several more times, until they decided that they could not agree with some of the practices there. They then encouraged the Seventh-day Adventist organization to build its own health-treatment facility.

It is evident that the health-reform movement was well underway long before Mrs. White wrote on the subject. It is also evident that at least some of her health concepts significantly resemble those that other reformers were advocating. The central question, then, is: Did Mrs. White receive her health message from God, or, as Numbers implies, from other (human) sources? Expressing this question in the language of research, we can say that we must test between two hypotheses:

Prophetess of Health, by Ronald Numbers

C1 Ellen G. White's health concepts can be satisfactorily explained as borrowed from the other health reformers of her day.

C2 Ellen G. White's health writings contain information that cannot be explained as arising from health concepts available in her day; they show she must have received information from an extrahuman source.

What type of evidence must we have to test these hypotheses? Does *Prophetess of Health* contain the necessary evidence? The researcher will need to gather the evidence in a way that neutralizes possible bias. Doing so will require carefully developing a list of all health principles that nineteenth-century health reformers, including Ellen White, advocated. To be meaningful, the list must be complete and not include just the principles that the researcher finds interesting or that support his or her favorite hypothesis.

Once we have this list, we can then compare it with each health-reform publication to determine a couple of things: (1) which items overlap on the lists from the different reformers, and (2) considering the publication dates, which health principles could possibly have been borrowed from a previous reformer. To avoid bias in the process of data collection, the researcher must use the same method in compiling each reformer's list of principles. Then we'll want some way to determine the relative correctness of those principles. We'll want to know if Mrs. White used principles unknown to the other reformers that have proven to be true—or at least if she chose a higher percentage of correct principles than the others, showing a better source of information. Or does the evidence suggest that she "borrowed" principles from the other reformers guided only by her own human wisdom?

How do we assess the accuracy of these health principles? We can judge them by current medical knowledge, but our modern knowledge, in spite of its amazing improvement in recent decades, is not absolute and could be wrong in some cases. However, that may not be a serious problem for our research project. Medical science *has* improved tremendously, and as long as our twenty-first-century judgment of nineteenth-century health principles is usually reliable, and as long as we evaluate all the nineteenth-century reformers' writings using the same standard, we can arrive at a satisfactory conclusion as to the *relative* correctness of each reformer's health principles. We can't say for sure that a reformer was 100 percent correct or 76 percent or 32 percent, but we *can* determine if reformer X was correct substantially more often than reformer Y. This should provide a sufficient test of our two hypotheses. In the next chapter we'll examine the evidence for ourselves. For now, however, let's look at four objections to Ron Numbers's work.

Four Objections

First, Ron Numbers used neither the research method described above nor an acceptable alternative to it that would have allowed him to reach objective conclusions. On the positive side, he appears to have made a careful study of the history of nineteenth-century health reform. His book tells us when the reformers published their works, and it describes some health concepts they advocated. However, it provides a very incomplete picture of the health principles that Mrs. White and the other reformers advocated and gives no indication of what guidelines (if any) he followed in choosing what to include and what to leave out.

Numbers seems to have chosen a particular set of data on which to base his book. Instead of making a comparison of all of White's health ideas with those of others of her day and of ours, he seems to have selected the health concepts she advocated that other health reformers in her day also advocated. But emphasizing the similarities and ignoring the differences is not a valid methodology. The research presented in the next chapter will analyze how much overlap there was and how her health principles differed from those of the other reformers.

Second, Numbers's evaluation of the relationship between Ellen White's health concepts and those of the other reformers is also faulty in that he uses strictly *anecdotal evidence.* Imagine that I attend a lecture on healthful living and learn of a number of changes that I should make to improve the quality of my life. However, I respond that Uncle Bill smoked, drank a lot of alcohol, and ate very unhealthful food, and he was still lively when he died in a car accident at ninety-five years of age. "And," I say, "my neighbor Elmer had about the same results from a similar lifestyle, so those 'health nuts' don't know what they're talking about."

The problem with my thinking is that I have based my conclusion on limited data. I have forgotten about my other neighbor, Joe, who ate too much unhealthful food and died of a heart attack at age forty-six. If we examine a large, random sample of people, we find that some are born with strong bodies that will stand a lot of abuse, while others are not very strong genetically. We also find, significantly, that all—both the genetically lucky and the less fortunate—can improve their lifespan and quality of life by living healthfully.

A limited sample, like that of my Uncle Bill and neighbor Elmer, provides what is called anecdotal data, which means using only a few pieces of data that were not selected in a way that would make them objective and unbiased. Following this approach, we can easily produce data that fit our personal prejudices—like my unconsciously (or consciously!) choosing Uncle Bill and neighbor Elmer because their experience supports my own desire to avoid changing my lifestyle! We cannot trust anecdotal evidence to lead us to a valid conclusion.

Ron Numbers based his principal conclusions about Ellen White's inspiration on anecdotal evidence. His research design was completely inadequate to support the conclusions he made. Numbers implied that since in some ways Mrs. White's health concepts resembled those of others who were writing in her day, she must have copied from them. But the information included in

Prophetess of Health doesn't point incontrovertibly to this conclusion. We must evaluate Numbers's conclusion by determining the relative accuracy of Mrs. White's choice of health concepts.

Third, if we wish to use scholarly research to test a hypothesis, we cannot begin by assuming the hypothesis is false. This is circular reasoning and demonstrates nothing. However, Numbers seemed to do exactly this, because he didn't even try to evaluate objectively the hypothesis of divine inspiration. Rather, he started with the assumption that the data should be explained without recourse to that hypothesis. In the preface to *Prophetess of Health,* he stated this directly: "I have tried to be as objective as possible. Thus I have refrained from using divine inspiration as an historical explanation." Numbers may have felt that his evidence justified his rejection of divine input, but he didn't have the data to support this conclusion.

Fourth, Numbers devoted a significant part of his book to detailing some of Mrs. White's human frailties. From the late 1860s until at least the late 1880s there was considerable backsliding among Adventists on health reform. Apparently, on several occasions during those years, Mrs. White ate meat, becoming a strict vegetarian again only in 1894.[5] Does this undermine her claim of divine inspiration? Before her health visions, meat comprised a large part of her diet. After advocating vegetarianism, she struggled for many years to overcome her taste for meat. Should we be surprised at this? Should God have suddenly made her supernatural? It seems rather that God educated her over a period of time and that during that time she had to learn how to deal with her appetite for meat.

In *Spiritual Gifts,* which she wrote in 1864 after her main health vision, she cautioned against the use of phrenology.[6] However, not long after publishing *Spiritual Gifts,* during the White family's visit to Jackson's Home on the Hillside, she wrote enthusiastically to friends about Jackson's phrenological analysis of her sons. She was human, and apparently she didn't succeed in consistently practicing what she preached. We may have a hard time with this; we may expect her not to have exhibited the human weakness that the rest of us experience. But is it reasonable to think that God perfects the entire personal life and personal correspondence of those who serve as His inspired spokespersons? Perhaps, as we noted in chapter two, we should evaluate Mrs. White's work by studying her publications rather than the details of her private life.

Other Viewpoints

In 1976, the staff of the Ellen G. White Estate wrote *A Critique of Prophetess of Health,* a 127-page book responding to Numbers's book.[7] *A Critique* introduces many exhibits that Ron Numbers didn't cite and discusses information that seems to support an interpretation of Ellen White that differs from his. The book is long and detailed, and I won't attempt to summarize it here. I recommend reading it along with *Prophetess of Health* and comparing the two books. The White Estate critique provides information that helps one evaluate Numbers's conclusions, but it doesn't contain the kind of information that can settle the question of Mrs. White's inspiration. It's not the research project we're looking for.

In 2001, Dr. Mervyn Hardinge wrote a book that, while not intended to provide a comprehensive answer to *Prophetess of Health,* deals with some of the same questions. In this book, *A Physician Explains Ellen White's Counsels on Drugs, Herbs, and Natural Remedies,*[8] Dr. Hardinge examined the nature of health care, drugs, and medical education in the United States during the time Mrs. White was writing about health. He compared what others were saying with her counsel. So, while Hardinge didn't directly address many of the issues that Numbers raised, his book is relevant to our questions about the validity of Mrs. White's health counsel. The following summarizes Hardinge's findings.

Medical training during the 1800s was very meager. During the first part of the century, it consisted of merely an apprenticeship with a physician. There were no standards for this training, and quality varied considerably. By the 1880s some medical schools offered a two-year medical course. However, the second year repeated much of the content of the first year, and there were still no educational standards. More serious improvements were in evidence late in the century. By 1889, most medical schools gave a four-year program undergirded with basic science courses.

Medical practice during the 1800s was characterized by treatments aimed at symptoms, with no diagnosis of the real cause of the problem. Treatments were typically harsh and often dangerous. The prominent methods physicians used included inducement of vomiting and purging, blistering of the skin with noxious agents, extensive bloodletting, and the prescription of heavy doses of harsh and even poisonous drugs—strychnine, lead, mercury (calomel), antimony, iron, arsenic, hydrochloric acid, and manganese—that had no connection to the medical needs of the patients. It isn't hard to understand why the death rates of patients were so high, and why during that era the health reformers began to attract considerable attention by their opposition to conventional medical practices.

This context explains the statements Mrs. White made warning against the use of drugs to treat medical problems. She was not addressing her counsel against the use of modern drugs that treat specific physiological problems; she was warning about the harsh drugs listed above and especially about the focus on using high doses of these drugs instead of trying to improve people's health habits.

Dr. Hardinge's information doesn't provide a specific, rigorous test of whether Ellen White's health counsel requires a more-than-human source; it will take a different type of study to accomplish that. Hardinge's work does serve us by providing a better understanding of exactly what her health counsel meant and what medical practices she opposed. We'll misunderstand her counsel if we compare it with today's medical practices, because they differ greatly from the medical care available in her time. If we compare her counsel with nineteenth-century medicine, we'll understand it much better.

Mrs. White opposed the uninformed, dangerous medical care of that time and advocated simple remedies aimed at supporting the human body's healing mechanisms. When we study all her counsel, we see that she did not take extreme positions. She sometimes even used and recommended strong drugs when "wisely administered," but she cautioned that people should use them sparingly, and healthful living should be a priority. Mrs. White differed from other reformers in that she also had the positive goal of transforming the teaching of physicians and nurses. As the twentieth century dawned, with its improvements in medical care, she was involved in the establishment of schools to train nurses and physicians.

When we see Ellen White's health principles in their nineteenth-century context, they impress us with their good sense. However, none of the authors we have discussed so far has provided evidence that we can use to test the two hypotheses detailed above, C1 and C2. In the next chapter we'll look at a serious attempt to test these hypotheses.

---

1. Ronald Numbers, *Prophetess of Health: A Study of Ellen G. White* (New York: Harper & Row, 1976).

2. See S. I. McMillen, *None of These Diseases* (Grand Rapids, Mich.: Fleming H. Revell, 1984). Also summarized from Numbers's book.

3. Numbers, 80, 81.

4. Ellen G. White, "Questions and Answers," *Advent Review and Sabbath Herald*, No. 17 (October 8, 1867), 30:260.

5. Numbers, 169–174.

6. Ellen G. White, *Spiritual Gifts* (Hagerstown, Md.: Review and Herald, 1945), 4:80.

7. *A Critique of Prophetess of Health* (Silver Spring, Md.: The Ellen G. White Estate, 1976).

8. Mervyn Hardinge, *A Physician Explains Ellen White's Counsels on Drugs, Herbs, and Natural Remedies* (Hagerstown, Md.: Review and Herald, 2001).

CHAPTER 5

The Test

The Seventh-day Adventist Church has proclaimed a message on healthful living since the mid-1800s. The content and influence of this message arose from the prophetic role of Ellen White. Whom should we now trust—Mrs. White or those who have challenged the claim that her health message was God-given?

On one hand:

- Mrs. White's writings have produced one of the longest-lived large groups of people.
- The principles she enunciated accurately parallel modern thinking about lifestyle.

On the other hand:

- Mrs. White made health and medical statements that medical science has not been able to verify.
- Many of her health principles are found in the works of others who wrote before her and concurrent with her.

A couple of Bible texts give us a place to begin searching for the answer:

> If what a prophet proclaims in the name of the Lord does not take place or come true, that is a message that the

> Lord has not spoken. That prophet has spoken presumptuously. Do not be afraid of him (Deuteronomy 18:22).

> Watch out for false prophets. They come in sheep's clothing, but inwardly they are ferocious wolves. By their fruit you will recognize them. Do people pick grapes from thornbushes, or figs from thistles? Likewise every good tree bears good fruit, but a bad tree bears bad fruit. A good tree cannot bear bad fruit, and a bad tree cannot bear good fruit. Every tree that does not bear good fruit is cut down and thrown into the fire. Thus, by their fruit you will recognize them (Matthew 7:15–20).

These texts make it clear: We can expect to hear both from good prophets who speak for God and from false prophets whom God has not inspired. God has given us the right and in fact the responsibility to distinguish between them. The test is their "fruit"—the accuracy of what they have said or written. We are not being presumptuous when we challenge the work of Ellen White and examine it for accuracy, because God has asked us to discriminate between genuine and false prophets. If Ellen White's health principles are from God, the evidence will verify that.

Modern scholarship has challenged the concept of "prophet" at another level as well. Biblical prophets claim that God spoke to them and gave them information—propositional truths. While the prophets seem to have recorded this information in their own words and writing style, they claimed that the concepts came from God. However, many modern scholars deny this supernatural communication of actual information. In their view, God may in some way stimulate prophets to write on some subject, but He doesn't give them any concrete information. What the prophets write is of human, not divine, origin. This orientation seems to be at least part of the basis for Ron Numbers's statement in the preface of *Prophetess of Health*: "I have tried to be as objective as possible.

Thus I have refrained from using divine inspiration as an historical explanation."

I suggest that when one is judging between true and false prophets, objectivity means not assuming that divine inspiration either *was* or *was not* involved. Rather, it means using a careful research methodology to test the hypothesis of divine inspiration, divine communication. We must describe our objective for such a test carefully. It's not likely that we can prove that divine communication was involved. We can, however, test the hypothesis that "some type of supernatural communication is needed to explain what the prophet has written." If we can demonstrate that the prophet had access to ordinary human resources that can adequately account for the information delivered in his or her message, then we have refuted or at least seriously weakened the hypothesis that "supernatural communication is needed."

However, merely showing that the other health reformers of Ellen White's day were publishing many or even all of the health principles she promoted will not refute the hypothesis of supernatural communication. The possibility exists that God intended the entire health-reform movement of the 1800s to pave the way for Ellen White's health message. To have a valid test, we must also compare the relative correctness of the health principles she promoted to that of the other reformers' principles. If her message is no more correct than theirs is, then it would appear that the hypothesis of divine communication has been refuted. But if significantly more of her principles are correct, then her correctness will require an explanation.

As we noted in the previous chapter, we do not have an absolute standard of medical truth to use in making this test. However, this is not a serious problem. Comparison with modern medical knowledge will be an adequate test because we need to determine just the *relative* correctness of Ellen White's principles compared with that of the other health reformers' principles. If comparison with modern concepts incorrectly judges some of her health principles, it will also incorrectly judge the other health reformers in the same way.

If Ellen White received divine insight into health principles, her writings will stand the test of comparison with medical knowledge. If she borrowed her health ideas and if human knowledge is sufficient to explain her choices, then we would have shown that divine communication was not required. In that case, we would just have to say the evidence is not adequate to test the source of her information. (God could use a prophet to bring the works of another author to our attention. In that case, we wouldn't have the evidence to determine whether divine communication was involved.)

Another possible test is the relative health of those who live by her health principles compared with those who don't. If the followers of her principles are healthier, that also requires an explanation. We will discuss this approach first.

The Health of Adventists

During the first half of the twentieth century, up to the late 1950s, medical and nutritional knowledge made Adventist health principles seem like an unfortunate mistake. For example, nutritionists considered a vegetarian diet very inadequate for maintaining good health. Since that time, research in medical and nutritional science has increased greatly, and it has reversed this opinion. Medical authorities now regard the Adventist lifestyle as the epitome of desirable lifestyles.

In 1958, Loma Linda University initiated a massive research project called the Adventist Health Study. This study compared the health of Seventh-day Adventist Californians with the health of the general population of California. Many members of the Adventist Church follow Ellen White's health principles and seem to be healthier because of it. Researchers began the Adventist Health Study to determine whether this seeming health advantage is a reality and to document how specific principles of healthful living affect our health.

Recent findings of this study indicate that the average California Adventist man can expect to live 7.3 years longer than the average non-Adventist California man does. Adventist California women live 4.4 years longer than their non-Adventist counterparts do. For vegetarian Adventists, the difference in life expectancy is 9.5 years for men and 6.1 years for women. The study also compared California Adventists with life expectancy data for the entire United States and nine other countries, and California Adventists seem to be the longest-lived group of all.[1]

All the following factors contributed to increased longevity for men and women: vegetarian diet, exercise, eating nuts, controlling weight, and refraining from smoking. The vegetarian Adventists not only live longer than nonvegetarian Adventists do, they are also healthier, with a significantly lower risk of colon cancer and, for men, a lower risk of prostate cancer and of fatal heart disease. (The latter is not as clear for women.) The vegetarian Adventists also seem to have a lower risk of developing diabetes mellitus, hypertension, and arthritis.[2]

Does the distinctly better health and greater longevity of the followers of Ellen White's health principles prove that she was the recipient of divine communication? *Prove* is a very big word and must always be used with caution. One could propose a variety of explanations for at least part of this phenomenon, and we'd need to examine them against the evidence. For example, perhaps the explanation is not that Ellen White's health principles were exceptional. Perhaps, instead, she is very influential in the lives of Seventh-day Adventists, leading many of them to value good health more highly than do other portions of the population. In that case, though, a question would remain: Why did it take one hundred years for medical science to come around to confirming the principles that Ellen White advocated? What is the likelihood that she would have known in the nineteenth century health principles that medical science now understands but that were unknown as recently as the 1950s? That seems unlikely. However, to test the hypothesis of divine communication, we still need more specific evidence on the quality and origin of Ellen White's health principles. Fortunately, someone has dug up that evidence.

A Striking New Analysis

Don McMahon, M.B.B.S., F.R.A.C.S., D.L.O. (the Australian equivalent of an American M.D. plus postgraduate degrees), has completed a comparison of Ellen White's health principles with her supposed sources and with modern medical principles.* What follows in most of the rest of this chapter is based on his research and is presented from his point of view.

* * * * *

When I was in medical school in the late 1950s, one of the teachers assigned the other students and me to record what we ate during a two-week period. I was following the Adventist lifestyle, so I was a lacto-ovo-vegetarian (a vegetarian who also eats eggs and dairy products). Of course, the record I kept during those two weeks reflected my eating habits. The lecturer singled me out in class as having a very inadequate diet, and other students sent a considerable amount of "friendly" ridicule my way.

Since that time, medical and nutritional knowledge has increased greatly, reversing opinions as to what constitutes a desirable lifestyle. On the twenty-fifth anniversary of my graduation, I went to a reunion of my medical class. A number of my former classmates apologized to me for the ridicule, saying they had adopted many features of my lifestyle and were advocating the same to their patients. Several asked me how I had known these health principles so many years before they were known to science.

This episode encouraged me to make a detailed study of the health principles in the writings of Ellen White. Preparation for

---

*A report of McMahon's research is available in his book *Acquired or Inspired? Exploring the Origins of the Adventist Lifestyle* (Warburton, Australia: Signs Publishing Co., 2005). A CD detailing McMahon's research accompanies the book.

this task came partly from a previous writing project: I wrote a series of fifty-two articles on health, each article presenting one health principle illustrated with a few physiological statements and some epidemiology or pathogenesis. In preparing to write these articles, I had carefully studied medical journal articles on lifestyle and health.

After completing this writing project, I re-read Ellen White's *Ministry of Healing*[3] and found nearly all of the fifty-two health principles there. The health principles she recommended in that book—what practices people should follow—are consistent with modern medical knowledge. But the physiological explanation she gave of these principles—why these practices work—often do not accord with modern physiology. This experience led to the following study, which seeks to assess the overall accuracy or correctness of Ellen White's health writings.

Research Method

Beginning in 1848, Ellen White wrote many articles and comments on health, including statements that appeared again in her book *The Ministry of Healing*. I extracted all the health and medical statements I could find in this book. I traced most of these statements back to the original source in her writings to see if and how she had altered them in later uses. (I rarely found more than slight alteration in the wording. I did find a few fundamental changes that followed new medical knowledge accumulating in her day.) I extracted each health and medical statement in the health section of her book *Spiritual Gifts* in the same way.

I assigned each of Ellen White's health or medical statements to one of two categories: "whats" and "whys." A "what" is a statement of a lifestyle principle; a statement of what to do or not do to remain healthy—for example, "don't eat meat," or "drink lots of water." A "why" is an explanation of the reason for a "what" principle—usually a physiological statement explaining why the lifestyle principle is valid.

There is good evidence that Ellen White saw the difference between health principles and the explanations for them. For example, she wrote,

> I use some salt, and always have, because from the light given me by God, this article, in the place of being deleterious, is actually essential for the blood. The whys and wherefores of this I know not, but I give you the instruction as it is given me.[4]

She always distinguished between physiology on the one hand ("whys"), and hygiene or health reform on the other hand ("whats"). She saw the former as community knowledge that should be taught in government schools and the latter as special knowledge that Adventist families should teach.[5]

I judged the accuracy of each of Ellen White's health and medical statements as compared with my personal knowledge of modern medical opinion derived from my study of medical research journals. When her statements used words no longer used or with a different meaning in modern usage, before scoring her statement I sought the meaning of these words at the time of her writing, either in the context or from other contemporary health writings.

I gave each of her statements a score of one if I considered it to have been verified or zero if not. (If modern medical research has supported the truth of the health principle, I considered it "verified"; but if modern medical research has not yet supported the principle, I considered it "unverified.") Then I calculated a total score and a percentage score for all such statements in a given book.*

---

*In evaluating the correctness of Ellen White's statements, we must understand the historical context in which she gave them. Unless we do, we might seriously misinterpret some of them. For example, she condemned the use of arsenic, strychnine, and quinine, grouping the three together. Critics often cite this as a seriously false medical statement, because quinine is an important treatment for malaria. To understand her correctly, we must recognize that when she made this statement, quinine was not used specifically for malaria. It was given in large doses to anyone who had a fever. Later, she approved its use specifically for malaria.

In addition, three other Seventh-day Adventist medical practitioners who are also well acquainted with modern medical research in lifestyle and health scored her work in the same way. The scoring by the different individuals varied somewhat. In the scoring of statements in *The Ministry of Healing*, there was a variation of 15 percent between the highest and lowest score. My score was about in the middle of this range. I considered my scores a reasonable average of all the scores, and so I used them in the results I report here.

Further, I categorized each "what" statement that I considered verified as to its significance for health. Thus, in some of the analyses, I placed each principle in one of three categories: (1) unverified, (2) verified and minor, or (3) verified and significant. A "minor" principle is one that is correct but will only have a minor effect on health, whereas a "significant" principle will have a prominent, positive effect on health. Again, I based my categorization of a health practice as "minor" or "significant" on evaluations of the risk factors of these practices published in the medical literature.

In the research results given below, I have categorized statements as "verified" or "unverified" and as "minor" or "significant." Please remember that these categorizations are not based on an absolute standard. Rather, they are my judgments based on current medical knowledge.

I also analyzed and scored the health writings of several of the most prominent health reformers of Ellen White's era—works she knew—in the same way. I did this to the publications of Sylvester Graham, William Alcott, Larkin Coles, James Caleb Jackson, and John Harvey Kellogg. I scored Ellen White's works fairly hard, and I scored all the others by the same standard because I believe doing so results in a fair comparison.

"Whats" and "Whys"

My research began with a study of *The Ministry of Healing*. After collecting all the health and medical statements, I divided the statements into "whats" and "whys" categories and then further divided the correct "what" statements into "minor" and "significant" categories. Consideration of the timing of Ellen White's health visions, her writing out of the information given in the visions, and her statements about when she began reading the works of other health reformers led me to the next step of my study: a comparison of her writings with the writings of other health reformers of her day.

Ellen White's most significant health vision occurred in June 1863. Soon after this, she wrote a brief summary of the vision, originally published in 1863.[6] A more complete presentation of the health principles of the 1863 vision appeared in *Spiritual Gifts* in the summer of 1864. Mrs. White stated, "I did not read any works upon health until I had written *Spiritual Gifts.*"[7] She further said that after writing the *Spiritual Gifts* statement she began reading the publications of other health reformers and using some of their material to show how closely it followed what God had shown her. She wrote, "I then searched the various works on hygiene and was surprised to find them so nearly in harmony with what the Lord had revealed to me. And to show this harmony, and to set before my brethren and sisters the subject as brought out by able writers, I determined to publish 'How to Live,' in which I largely extracted from the works referred to."[8] To evaluate the influence that these health reformers had on her, I analyzed their publications for comparison with her material.*

Before I present the results of this research, let's consider three possible outcomes and what each would mean. All three recognize that Ellen White had no medical education at the time she wrote her health principles.

D1 If she was deceived in thinking God had given her a revelation, then the health principles ("whats") in *Spiritual*

*In the CD that accompanies *Acquired or Inspired?*, I have described all of these stages in the research in the order in which I did them, to show how each step in the analysis revealed the need for the next step. In this book I'll give just the results.

Gifts should be essentially nonsense. And when she began reading the works of other reformers and incorporating their ideas, the level of correctness of her statements should increase to match theirs.

D2 If she copied her health principles from the other reformers with no divine input, the correctness of her statements in *Spiritual Gifts* will match the level of correctness of those reformers, and her subsequent health writings should improve in correctness only as much as her sources improve.

D3 If the "whats" in *Spiritual Gifts* resulted from genuine inspiration—from divinely revealed information—they should display a high correctness level. This correctness level should then decline as she began to read the works of other reformers and to use their material (which she said she did).

Spiritual Gifts contains forty-six "what" statements, and I considered forty-four (96 percent) of these to be verified, with 70 percent being significant principles and 26 percent minor (see figure 5.1). In *The Ministry of Healing,* Mrs. White added forty more "whats" to those she had included in *Spiritual Gifts.* (Several *Spiritual Gifts* "whats" are not found in *The Ministry of Healing.*) Of these forty extra principles, I considered thirty-one (78 percent) to be verified, with only 40 percent significant and 38 percent minor (see figure 5.1). This result is consistent with the predictions of the inspiration model above (D3).

The correctness level of the "whys" in these books differs considerably from that of the "whats." *Spiritual Gifts* contains only twenty-six "whys," with ten (38 percent) verified. *The Ministry of Healing* contains an extra fifty-two "whys," with twenty-five (48 percent) verified. (See figure 5.2.) Ellen White's "whats" have a high level of correctness, but her "whys" are no more correct than are those of the other reformers. Furthermore, the level of correctness of the "whys" changed in the opposite direction from

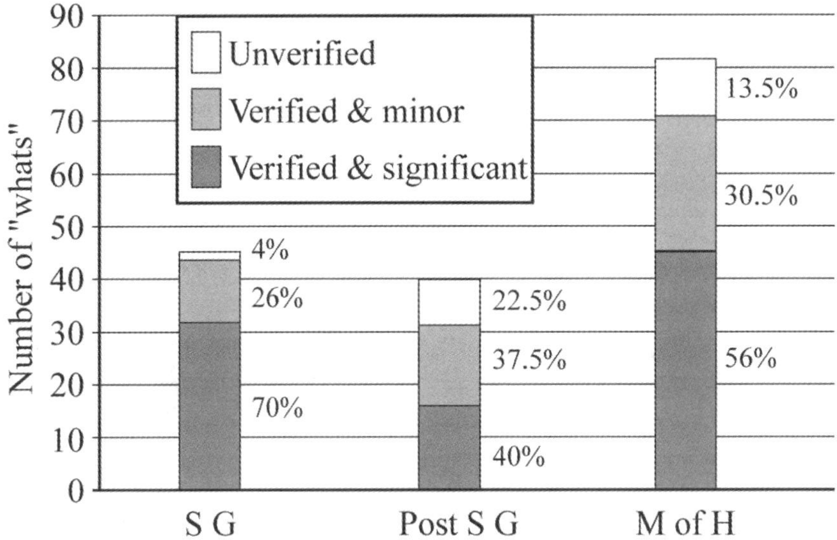

Figure 5.1. Number and percentage of "whats" (health principles) in three categories, in two Ellen White publications

In this and each of the following figures, the height of each shaded portion of the bars indicates the number of "whats," and the numbers beside the bars indicate the percentage of "whats" in each category within the bars. "Verified"/"unverified" indicates whether modern science supports these "whats," and "minor"/"significant" refers to the author's assessment of their relative impact on health. (S G = *Spiritual Gifts*; Post S G = Ellen White publications after *Spiritual Gifts* but before *The Ministry of Healing*; M of H = *The Ministry of Healing*)

that of the "whats." The "whats" decreased in correctness after she began reading other health-reform publications, but that of the "whys" increased. These results for the "whys" follows the predictions of the copying model above (D2). Apparently, the "whats" and the "whys" came from different sources. We'll discuss the significance of this after we evaluate some additional evidence.

Jackson's Diphtheria Article

In February 1863, James White published in the *Review and Herald* an article by Jackson on treating diphtheria. Ellen White

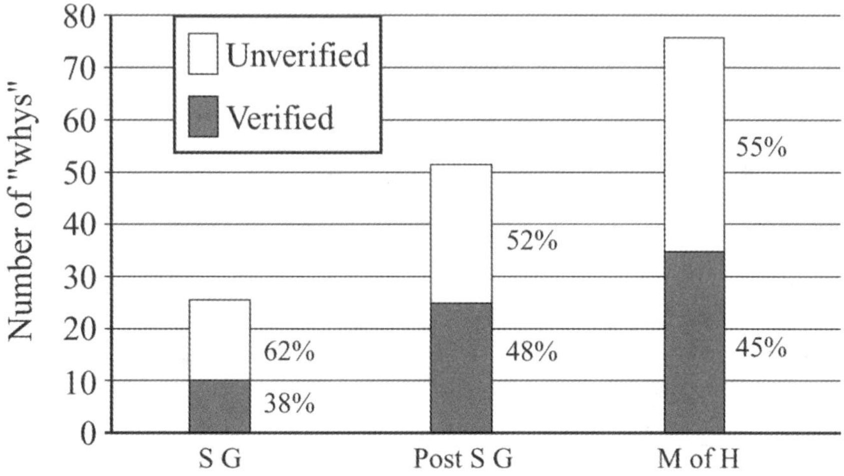

Figure 5.2. Number and percentage of "whys" (physiological explanations) in two categories in two Ellen White publications and post-*Spiritual Gifts* (See explanation in figure 5.1 caption.)

used the method of treatment described in this article to care for her sons when they contracted this disease. Since this occurred before her 1863 vision, some critics have claimed that she used Jackson's article as the basis for her *Spiritual Gifts* health principles. Other articles on health written by various health reformers were published in the *Review and Herald* in the few years before *Spiritual Gifts* (mostly in 1863 and early 1864); these also must be considered as possible sources for her health principles. So, I studied and scored all *Review and Herald* health articles from 1861 to mid-1864.

Jackson's article on diphtheria contained seventeen "whats"; only three of them appear among the twelve "whats" Ellen White used in her summary of the 1863 vision and in *Spiritual Gifts*. This rules out the possibility that Mrs. White based her health principles on the diphtheria article. An analysis of all the *Review and Herald* health articles up to June 6, 1863, reveals the same picture. Only five "whats" from these articles appear in the twelve "whats" in Ellen White's summary. And the percent of verified "whats" is much higher in the White summary than in the *Review*

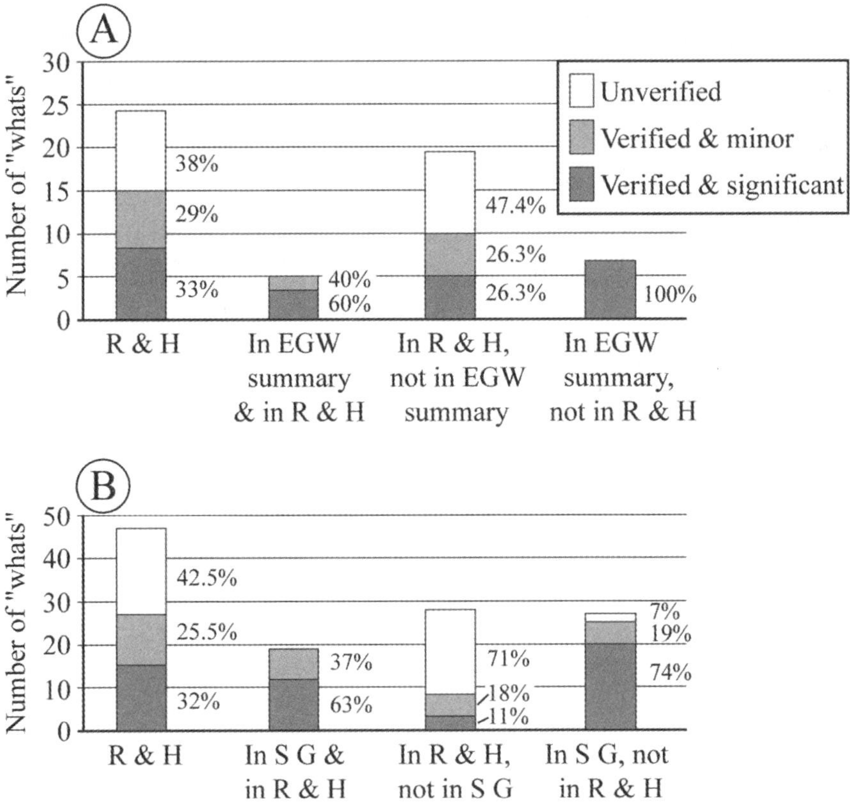

Figure 5.3. Number and percentage of "whats" in several publications

A. All health articles published in the *Review and Herald* (R & H) from 1861 to June 6, 1863 (the date of Ellen White's major health vision)

The bar labeled "In EGW summary & in R & H" shows the number of "whats" in Ellen White's brief summary in *Selected Messages*—which she wrote shortly after the June 1863 vision—that had also been published in *Review and Health* articles previous to that date. The bar labeled "In R & H, not in EGW summary" shows the number of "whats" that had been published in the *Review and Herald* that Ellen White did not include in her summary. The final bar, "In EGW summary, not in R & H" shows the number of additional "whats" Ellen White added in her summary that had not been published in the *Review and Herald.*

B. All *Review and Herald* health articles published from 1861 to mid-1864 (the time when the health section of *Spiritual Gifts* was written)

The bars show the same type of comparisons as in A above, but comparing the *Spiritual Gifts* material with previous *Review and Herald* publications.

and Herald articles (see figure 5.3A). In fact, the "whats" in Ellen White's material were 100 percent correct, while I judged as verified only 52 percent of the "whats" that were in the *Review and Herald* articles but that Ellen White didn't include in what she wrote.

The same picture emerges from a comparison of all the *Review and Herald* health articles to mid-1864 with Ellen White's list in *Spiritual Gifts,* written in the summer of 1864 (figure 5.3B). The fact that so few of the health principles in Mrs. White's early health publications appear also in the other articles falsifies the claim that she derived her health concepts from the *Review and Herald* articles.

There is another reason to discount the *Review and Herald* as her source. Ellen White included physiological explanations ("whys") for her health "whats." We would expect that if she had used the *Review and Herald* as a source, she would also use a good number of the *Review and Herald*'s "whys" in her writings. In fact, however, she used virtually none of the physiological "whys" found in the *Review and Herald.* Apparently, either she did not read the *Review and Herald* as she prepared her health principles for publication or she ignored it.

Now, let's compare the works of other nineteenth-century health reformers with Ellen White's health writings. We know that she read the publications of other health reformers—at least after writing *Spiritual Gifts.* Her copies of these books contain her underlining and other markings. In addition, sometimes she used the wording found in these other reform publications in her own works. This occurs often enough to indicate clearly that she was familiar with them and that they influenced her wording as she wrote. The bigger question is whether they were the source of her health principles or at least seriously influenced her choice of what principles to include in her writings.

Several health books, including Jackson's *The Laws of Life,*[9] were in the White household even before Ellen White wrote *Spiritual*

Gifts, but she stated that she did not read them until after writing out what she had seen in vision. It seems that at least James White read them, as he published a section of *Laws of Life* verbatim as an article in the *Review and Herald* on October 27, 1863. It's unlikely that Ellen White used these books as a source, however, because there is a dramatic difference in the correctness of the health principles in *Laws of Life* and *Spiritual Gifts* (see figure 5.4). Jackson's books contained numerous unverified principles, but Ellen White used almost none of them in her writings. In addition, she added twenty "whats" that were not in Jackson's books, and all of them have been verified! If we are going to be objective, we have to recognize that she had access to a much more accurate source of information than was available to Jackson. Her health principles did not come from Jackson's *Laws of Life*.

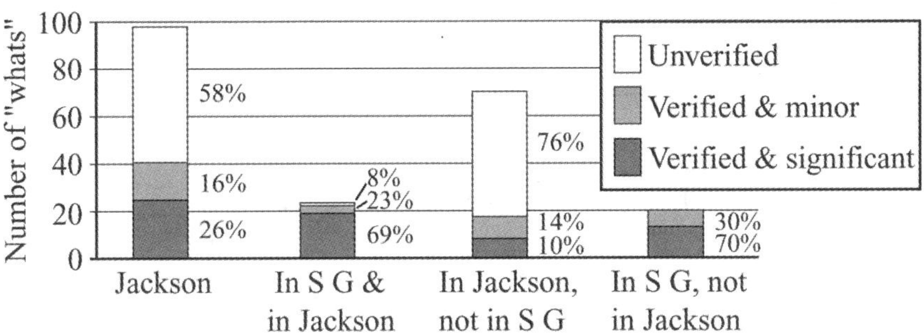

Figure 5.4. Comparison of health "whats" in the writings of Jackson and White

The last three bars show (1) the number of "whats" that both sources contain, (2) the number that Jackson used but White didn't, and (3) the "whats" White used that Jackson didn't.

Significantly More Are Correct

The works of several other health reformers were also in Ellen White's library, and she was familiar with them. These included publications of Sylvester Graham (early 1850s), William Alcott (1860), and Larkin B. Coles (1860). Evaluating each of these publications individually and comparing them with *Spiritual Gifts* and

The Ministry of Healing yields a similar picture to the one we have just seen with Jackson (see figure 5.5). Significantly more of the health principles Ellen White chose are correct than are those of any of the others.

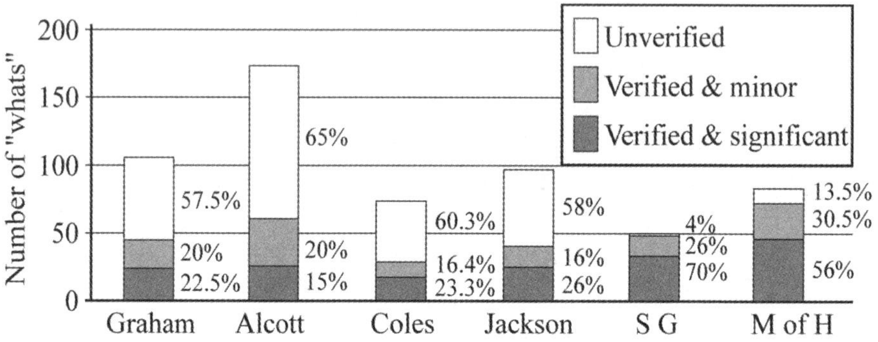

Figure 5.5. Comparison of health "whats" in the writings of four health reformers with the "whats" in *Spiritual Gifts* (S G) and *The Ministry of Healing* (M of H)

On what basis, then, could it be said that she borrowed her health message from the other reformers? Since she was largely uneducated and certainly had no medical training at all, how did she know which health principles to choose and which to ignore? And where did she get the extra "whats" that are not found in the writings of other reformers but that have been verified? True divine inspiration is one explanation. Does anyone have another realistic explanation?

Ron Numbers placed side by side a couple paragraphs from Mrs. White and very similar paragraphs from Coles regarding meat-eating. He concluded:

> In view of Ellen White's indignant assertions that her testimonies were not subject to human influences—"I am as dependent upon the Spirit of the Lord in writing my views as I am in receiving them"—her manifest reliance on Coles is, to say the least, puzzling.[10]

This statement illustrates the unreliability of the method used by Numbers and others. Basing an evaluation of Ellen G. White's inspiration on similarities of wording between her writings and other publications doesn't work. She made use of the wording from other publications in writing her own material, but my research makes it clear that she did not rely on these other health reformers as a source of lifestyle principles (see figure 5.5).

Added together, all the lifestyle principles that Graham, Alcott, Coles, and Jackson used (GACJ in figure 5.6) total three hundred health "whats." Two hundred eight (69 percent) of these are unverified. In contrast, *The Ministry of Healing* has a very high percentage of verified "whats." This book contains sixty "whats" that at least one of the other reformers used and that, consequently, one could claim that Ellen White borrowed. That claim has little meaning when we consider that of these sixty possibly borrowed "whats," only nine (15 percent) are unverified.

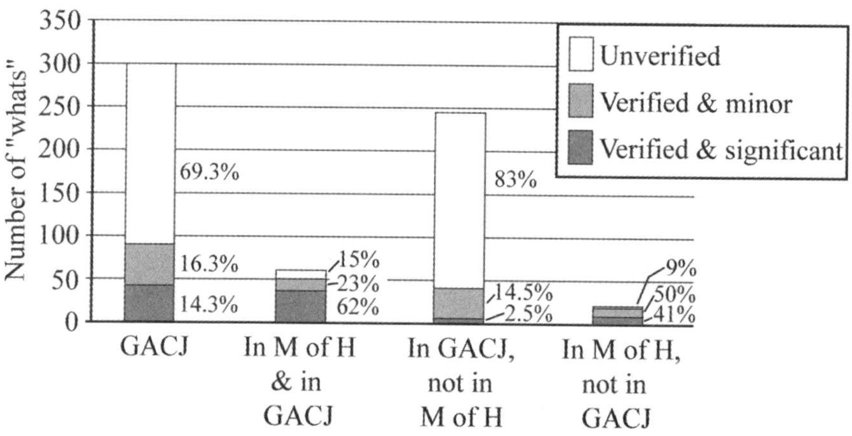

Figure 5.6. Comparison of the combined total of 300 health "whats" used by Graham, Alcott, Coles, and Jackson (GACJ), with those used by White in *The Ministry of Healing*

The last three bars show (1) the number of "whats" in *The Ministry of Healing* that were used by at least one of the other reformers, (2) the number used by at least one of the others but not used in *The Ministry of Healing*, and (3) additional "whats" in *The Ministry of Healing* that were not used by any of the other reformers.

Furthermore, Mrs. White added twenty-two additional "whats" that none of the other reformers used, and only two, or 9 percent, of these are unverified, whereas 199 (83 percent) of the 240 "whats" found in the writings of GACJ but not used by Mrs. White are unverified. Their low level of correctness is consistent with the meager medical knowledge of the 1800s. Ellen White's level of correctness, however, is profoundly inconsistent with any human source of medical information available anytime during the 1800s.

The level of correctness of the health principles Ellen White promoted stands out even more clearly when we compare the significant "whats" (see figure 5.6). Of the "whats" in *Ministry of Healing* that are also in GACJ, 62 percent are significant, but only 14 percent of the "whats" (forty-three of three hundred) in GACJ are significant. Nearly 250 "whats" in GACJ are not found in *Ministry of Healing*, and only six (3 percent) of these are significant. Of these six, Ellen White used four elsewhere in her writings; the only two she didn't use are "the need for air filters in factories" and "the avoidance of lead-based paints." Ellen White exhibited a phenomenal ability to recognize significant health principles and reject the nonsignificant ones. The other reformers did not have this ability.

What About Kellogg?

Ellen and James White encouraged a promising young student, John Harvey Kellogg, to attend medical school. Upon finishing, he worked closely with the Whites for some years. Ron Numbers stated that Kellogg supplied Ellen White with the latest medical information, and he insinuated that Kellogg's influence on Ellen White's medical principles "was not negligible."[11] So, it will be instructive to compare the record of his health teachings with hers.

Ellen White wrote *Spiritual Gifts* before Kellogg began his health education, so he couldn't have influenced the content of that material. In addition, sixty-four of the total eighty-two "whats" that Ellen White used in her writings were published before Kellogg entered medical school. So, obviously, he couldn't have influenced those health principles either. However, Mrs. White wrote *The Ministry of Healing* well after Kellogg graduated; thus, he could possibly have influenced the eighteen "new" principles in that book. We'll use *The Ministry of Healing* in our comparison with Kellogg (see figure 5.7).[12]

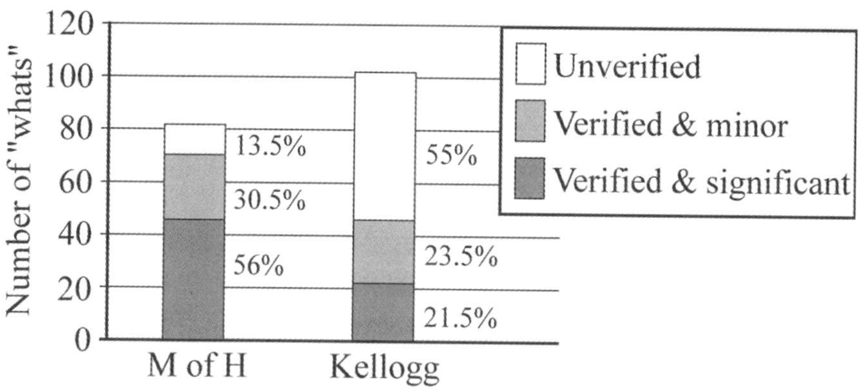

Figure 5.7. Comparison of the number of health "whats" in *The Ministry of Healing* with those published by Kellogg

Kellogg had a quality medical education and was a leading figure in late nineteenth-century medicine, writing extensively on lifestyle and health. However, his published lifestyle principles were 55 percent unverified, compared with the 13 percent unverified "whats" in *The Ministry of Healing*. Of the thirty-five "whats" that appear in both *The Ministry of Healing* and Kellogg's 1888 works, Mrs. White had published thirty-three before Kellogg was medically trained, and she published the other two (which others had already published) before 1888.

If we compare the correctness of Kellogg's principles with that of Graham, Alcott, Coles, and Jackson (figure 5.8A), it is evident that his are little improved over theirs. Even the percentage of correctness of Kellogg's physiological explanations for health principles ("whys" in figure 5.8B) is no higher than that of Jackson.

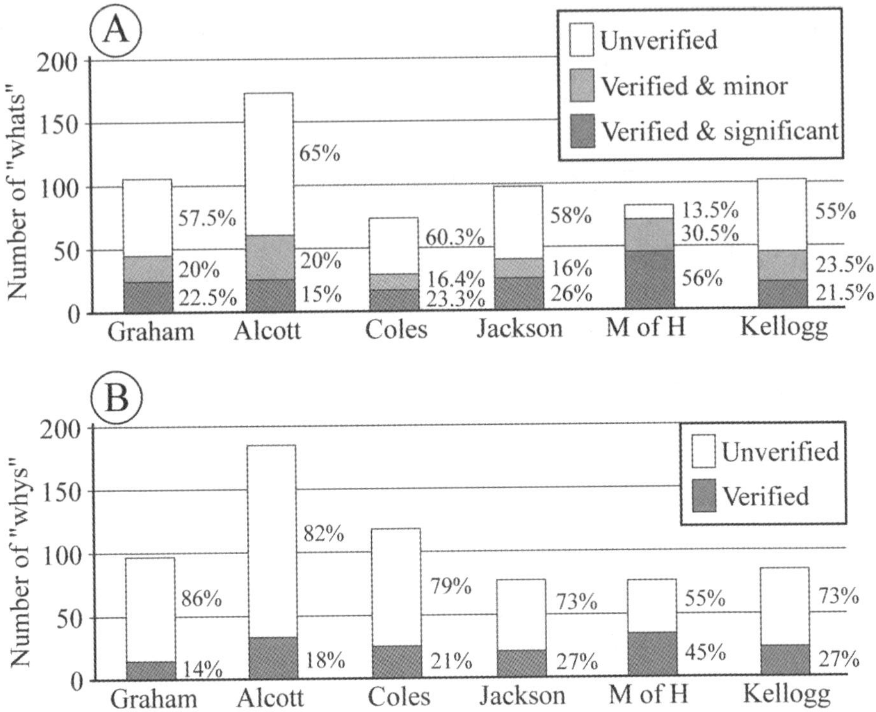

Figure 5.8. Comparison of the number of health "whats" (A) and "whys" (B) used in *The Ministry of Healing* with those used by five other reformers

More to the point, his "whats" compare very poorly with those of Mrs. White. Kellogg would have greatly improved his understanding of the principles of healthful living if he had borrowed more heavily from her and had ignored his other sources! The only "what" that Ellen White could have gotten from Kellogg was the concept that eating nuts is healthy. Kellogg included this principle in his 1899 medical text, and Ellen White first mentioned it in 1899.

Figure 5.9 makes another type of comparison. It conveys an analysis of whether some reformers improved on the record of those who wrote earlier and whether the early reformers could have been sources for the later reformers. Graham, who had no medical education, wrote years before Alcott, who was educated as a physician. Thus, we might expect Alcott to understand health

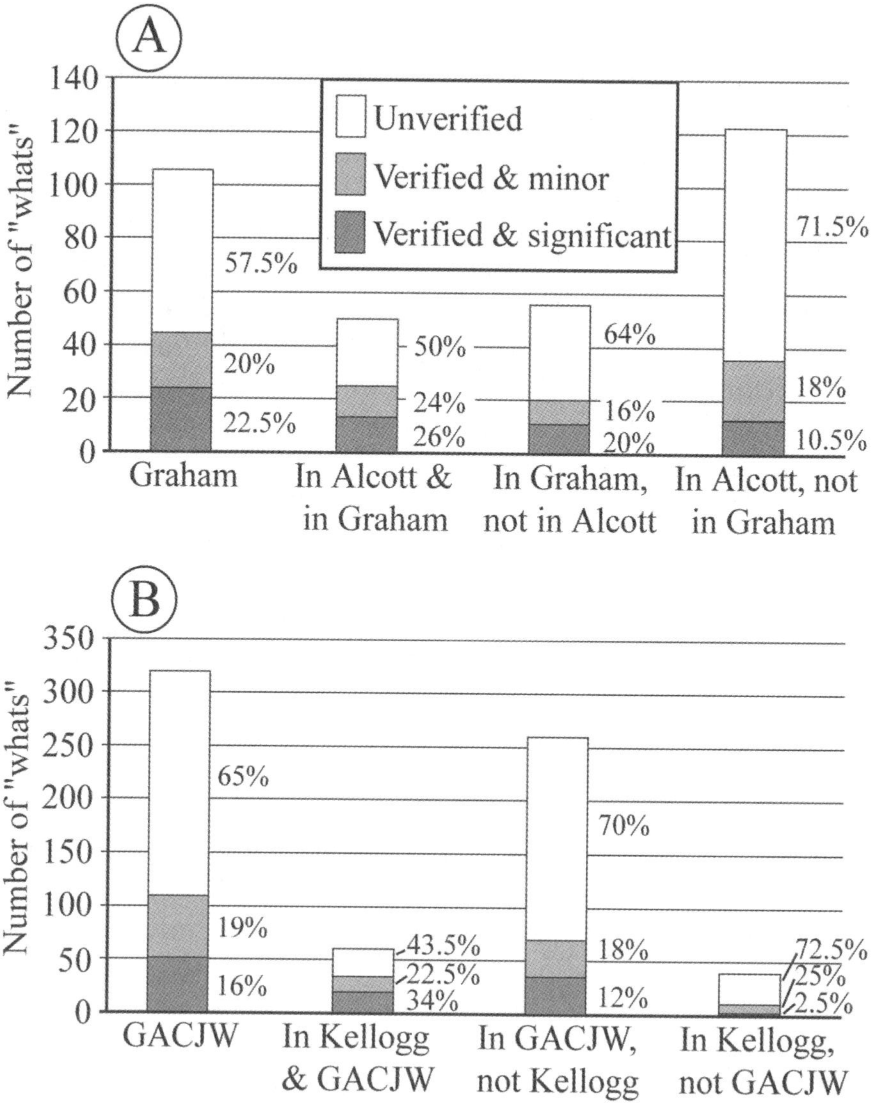

Figure 5.9. Comparisons showing the relative accuracy of the "whats" used by two health reformers as compared to the reformers who published before them

A. Alcott's writings compared with the earlier writings of Graham

B. Kellogg's writings compared with the combined total of "whats" used previously by Graham, Alcott, Coles, Jackson, and White (GACJW)

better than Graham did. Their levels of correctness don't support this expectation (see figure 5.9A). Of the "whats" in Graham that Alcott did not use, 64 percent are unverified—so Alcott did marginally better than chance in rejecting unverified concepts that Graham used. However, he diminished his level of correctness by adding 123 additional "whats" that are 72 percent unverified. If Alcott was using Graham as a source, he didn't improve on Graham's record even though he had a medical education. In contrast, if White used Graham as a source, she did make a very significant improvement over him in her choice of health principles despite her complete lack of any medical education. Making the same type of comparison between others of these reformers yields the same result.[13]

Our final comparison is between Kellogg and the combined "whats" of Graham, Alcott, Coles, Jackson, and White (GACJW in figure 5.9B). Kellogg could have obtained the writings of all these reformers, so it will be instructive to see if he, with his top quality medical education and reputation in health care, could improve on the record of the others. The "whats" that Kellogg and at least one of the others promoted are 44 percent unverified, which is a better record than the 65 percent unverified for GACJW. Of the 260 "whats" in GACJW that Kellogg did not use, 70 percent are unverified. So, Kellogg's record at choosing correct health principles was better than the combined record of the others. However, Kellogg spoiled that record by adding forty additional "whats" of his own that are 73 percent unverified.

It is instructive to divide Kellogg's "whats" into two groups: (1) those that are also in Ellen White's writings pre-1888, and (2) those that Kellogg had but that Ellen White didn't. It appears that Kellogg made a random selection of verified and unverified lifestyle principles from Mrs. White and a random selection of verified and unverified principles from the other reformers. Kellogg's level of correctness improves over the latter only because he used more "whats" from Ellen White than from the other reformers. Since this is true, and since the only "what" that Ellen White could have gotten from Kellogg is the principle of eating nuts, Numbers's statement that Kellogg's influence on Ellen White "was not negligible" is puzzling.

In 1895, Kellogg stated that Battle Creek Sanitarium kept five years ahead of the medical profession because when a new idea came from medical research, he would check it against Mrs. White's writings. If the new medical idea passed this test, he would begin using it immediately, but if the new idea didn't agree with her writings, he wouldn't use it. Thus, while other doctors were slowly evaluating the new medical ideas, Kellogg's use of Ellen White's counsel allowed him to move confidently ahead in the right direction.[14]

Spiritual Gifts "Whats"

We can consider the list of lifestyle principles in *Spiritual Gifts* to be the basic presentation of Ellen White's health message, since she wrote them soon after her 1863 vision, and they have the highest percentage of verified "whats." (See table 5.1—the tables appear on pages 76ff.) These principles, written in the era when microorganisms were first being discovered, are still an excellent guide to healthful living. I consider two of them unverified, but following these two principles would probably not cause any health problems. In contrast, the lists of "whats" advocated by other health reformers included some "health" principles that are rather strange or at least have no medical basis (see table 5.2). It is interesting that Ellen White did not pick up any of these and advocate them.

In addition, the "whats" added in *The Ministry of Healing* that were not also in *Spiritual Gifts* are mostly verified. Those that I consider unverified (see table 5.3) do not make the kind of serious health errors seen in table 5.2. Several items in table 5.3 do have some validity, but I did not consider them a sufficient health hazard to give them a positive score. Ellen White stated that after writing *Spiritual Gifts,* she read the writings of other health reformers and used some of their material. However, she still had a more balanced understanding of health principles than did these other reformers, and her accuracy level was far higher than theirs.

I scored one "what"—"don't eat blood"—with a zero. There may be objections to this since the Bible says we should not eat blood. The statement appears in this context: "No creature . . . from which the blood had not been carefully drained, could be used as food."[15] I could find no research that indicates the draining of blood from an animal at the time of slaughter decreases the risk of the meat. Nor do I know any reason why it should. The draining of blood at the time of slaughter doesn't eliminate all the blood. The flesh will always contain some blood; thus it will also contain any health risk the blood has. So, I had to give this principle a score of zero. We do not have access to any kind of absolute medical standard for scoring, and thus we cannot use current medical concepts to decide the absolute truth of health statements in the Bible or the writings of Ellen White. Our scoring method is only an imperfect but effective way to determine the *relative* accuracy of different health reformers.

I used statistical analysis to compare the difference between the levels of correctness of the "whats" promoted by Ellen White and those promoted by the other reformers.* Statistical analysis can tell us whether the differences are significant or can be explained by chance. It is clear that we can't realistically attribute the differences in correctness between Ellen White and the others to chance. The differences are large, they are very real, and they demand an explanation.

Let's return now to the two hypotheses from the previous chapter: (C1) Ellen G. White's health concepts can be satisfactorily explained as borrowed from the other health reformers of her day. (C2) Ellen G. White's health writings contain information that cannot be explained as arising from health concepts available in

*For the full statistical analysis, see *Acquired or Inspired?*

her day; she must have received information from an extra-human source. The results of this research have refuted hypothesis C1. We can't satisfactorily explain Ellen White's lifestyle principles by suggesting that she borrowed them from other health reformers. The data are consistent with hypothesis C2, which is that she must have had another source of health information.

Where did she get this better information? Must it have come from a nonhuman source? How did Ellen White know how to recognize valid concepts and reject the faulty ones? She had very little education of any kind and certainly no medical education. In any case, the medical education available then wouldn't have been helpful anyway. Divine inspiration best explains the data.

What About the "Whys"?

Ellen White's physiological explanations (figures 5.2, 5.8B) differ from the "whats." They do not have the high degree of correctness seen in the "whats." Her percentage of verified "whys" appears higher than that of any of the others (figure 5.8B), but this is an artifact. Physiological explanations ("whys") associated with verified "whats" would be more likely to be correct than would explanations associated with unverified "whats." If we compare only the "whys" associated with significant "whats" in Ellen White and the other reformers, we find that as many of their "whys" as hers are correct. It appears to me that the "whats" and the "whys" came from different sources of information. Perhaps God gave us the health principles to follow and left it for us to figure out the reasons why they work.

Indeed, He could not have explained some of the "whys" correctly at that time without inventing medical vocabulary and revealing physiological concepts that were not known until decades after Ellen White wrote. Even in a prescientific era, saying, "Don't eat meat," or "Drink lots of water," or "Get plenty of sleep" didn't require any special vocabulary or advanced knowledge. Anyone, then or now, could understand these instructions because they describe lifestyle choices that have remained essentially constant.

However, it would be another matter to explain the reasons for these instructions when no one knew about bacteria or viruses, to say nothing of our immune and endocrine systems. No human language even contained the words necessary to describe these systems and how they work.

Interestingly, when people are troubled by apparent medical errors that Ellen White made, it's usually the "whys" that trouble them. The Ellen White quotation that Numbers said she took directly from Coles is a series of "whys."[16] But the correctness, or lack thereof, of the "whys" is not a good test of whether Ellen White's health principles were inspired. It's her principles for living—the "whats"—that can affect our health. As long as we follow these principles, it doesn't matter whether or not we understand the physiological reasons for them—or even whether or not the reasons given, the "whys," are erroneous. It is evident that God has communicated the truths we need. It also is evident that the explanations He didn't communicate—which, in fact, He couldn't realistically communicate at that time—wouldn't affect our health anyway.

* * * * *

In this chapter you've read a summary of Don McMahon's research. Now I will suggest a more general application of concepts from that research. In Ellen White's descriptions of how she composed some of her other writings we can see parallels to the matter of the "whats" and "whys" in the health articles. In her introduction to *The Great Controversy*, she says that God revealed to her through visions how He interacted with events in human history. But, she says, He left her to study history books so that she could fill in the history to make a connected story.

Similarly, Moses told us the simple facts of creation but didn't explain how God did it. He told us what it is critical for us to understand—that God is the Creator, that we're created beings, that the Fall was the root of evil, and that we need a Savior. But we didn't need to understand how God could create a complex ecosystem of living things in seven days. We *couldn't* have understood it, so God didn't try to tell us.

These parallels help to explain why we should not be surprised at the difference in accuracy between the "whats" and "whys" of the health concepts. This difference need not weaken our confidence in the reliability of the "whats"—the principles of healthful living.

---

1. G. E. Fraser and D. J. Shavlik, "Ten Years of Life: Is It a Matter of Choice?" *Archives of Internal Medicine* (2001) 161:1645–1652.

2. See D. A. Snowdon, R. L. Phillips, and G. E. Fraser, "Meat Consumption and Fatal Ischemic Heart Disease," *Preventive Medicine* (1984), 13:490–500; P. K. Mills, W. L. Beeson, R. L. Phillips, and G. E. Fraser, "Cohort Study of Diet, Lifestyle, and Prostate Cancer in Adventist Men," *Cancer* (1989) 64:598–604; G. E. Fraser, T. M. Strahan, J. Sabate, W. L. Beeson, and D. Kissinger, "Effects of Traditional Coronary Risk Factors on Rates of Incident Coronary Events in a Low Risk Population: The Adventist Health Study," *Circulation* (1992) 86:406–413; and T. J. A. Key, G. E. Fraser, M. Thorogood, P. Appleby, V. Beral, G. Reeves, M. L. Burr, J. Chang-Claude, R. Frentzel-Beyme, J. W. Kuzma, J. Mann, and K. McPherson, "Mortality in Vegetarians and Non-Vegetarians: A Collaborative Analysis of 8,300 Deaths Among 76,000 Men and Women in Five Prospective Studies," *American Journal of Clinical Nutrition* (1998). For more details, see G. E. Fraser, *Diet, Life Expectancy, and Chronic Disease: Studies of Seventh-day Adventists and Other Vegetarians* (New York: Oxford University Press, 2003).

3. Ellen G. White, *The Ministry of Healing* (Nampa, Idaho: Pacific Press, 1905).

4. Ellen G. White, *Counsels on Diet and Foods* (Hagerstown, Md.: Review and Herald, 1946), 344.

5. See Ellen G. White, "Words to Christian Mothers: On the Subject of Life, Health, and Happiness," *Review and Herald,* October 31, 1871, 38:154, 155.

6. Ellen G. White, *Selected Messages* (Hagerstown, Md.: Review and Herald, 1980), 3:279.

7. Ellen G. White, "Questions and Answers," *Advent Review and Sabbath Herald,* October 8, 1867, 260.

8. Ibid.

9. Jackson, *The Laws of Life* (1862, 1863).

10. Numbers, 162, 163.

11. Numbers, 177, 178.

12. John Harvey Kellogg, *The Home Hand-Book of Domestic Hygiene and Rational Medicine* (London: International Tract Society, 1899).

13. See the McMahon CD that accompanies his book *Acquired or Inspired?*

14. White Estate Document File #269, cited in White Estate, 16, 17.

15. White, *Ministry of Healing,* 312.

16. Numbers, 162, 163.

Table 5.1. Health Principles ("Whats") in *Spiritual Gifts*
(categorized as to correctness and significance)

A. Verified and significant "whats"

Avoid:	Restrict:	Exercise
Drugs	Salt	Vegetable foods
Patent medicines	Butter	Whole-wheat flour
Secondhand tobacco smoke		Variety of food
	Moderate:	Clean water
Smoking	Milk	Plenty of water
Alcohol	Outdoors	Clean person
Hard drugs		Clean house
Meat	Daily and freely:	Clean clothes
Animal fat	Good lifestyle	Sanitation
Overeating	Ventilation	Trust in God
Idleness	Clean environment	Cheerfulness
	Sunlight	Willpower
	Recreation	

B. Verified and minor "whats"

Avoid:	When needed:	Daily and freely:
Hypnotism	Fasting	Simple foods
Phrenology	Adjust diet slowly	Soft water
Tea and coffee	Hydrotherapy	
Pig meat		
Spices		
Sleep after eating		
Wet house-building site		

C. Unverified "whats"

Avoid:	Usually:
Leaven in bread	Only two meals a day

Table 5.2. Unverified "Whats" From Other Health Reformers
(health advice that's contrary to modern science)

Sylvester Graham:
Don't heat your house
Go naked
Don't shave
Don't cut your hair
Don't use perfumes
Avoid strong odors—even pleasant ones, like the scent of flowers
Don't rock a baby to sleep
Don't use salt
If you must eat meat, eat it raw
Don't drink water—get your liquids only from fruit
Avoid activities that cause you to perspire

William A. Alcott:
Venesection (bleeding) has validity—e.g., for heart disease
Wear very little clothing, even when it's cold
Avoid excessive application of your mind
Reading light literature injures your health
Don't use eye glasses
Children shouldn't drop their voices in the midst of a sentence
Don't comfort children; crying is good for them
Don't protect your face or neck from subzero air
Avoid sweating in hot weather
Keep no plants in your bedroom
Don't nap during the day
Don't sleep in the same bed with someone else
Avoid excess pleasure or mental activity
Don't eat most vegetables other than potatoes
When eating meat, eat mostly the fat
Don't let children eat fruit
Overweight people are healthy people
Avoid eating breakfast

You needn't drink much; food provides nearly all the liquid you need
Wear coarse, rough clothing; it cleans the skin and reduces the need for bathing
Don't bathe early in the day

Larkin B. Coles:
Know your own phrenology
Avoid excessive spitting
Don't rock a child in a cradle
Don't eat cucumbers or some other vegetables
Don't talk while eating
Don't nurse babies at night
Avoid mental activity for an hour after eating
Sugar is good food
If you exercise, reduce the amount you eat
Drink little water
Bathe, preferably, in seawater
You needn't bathe more than once or twice a week

James C. Jackson:
A good lifestyle eliminates the need for vaccination
Don't wear black
Wear your hair long enough to cover your neck (advice for both sexes)
Marital sexual activity is dangerous to health
Phrenology is scientific
Children should avoid eating potatoes
You can live exclusively on bread
The best diet consists of grains and fruits alone
Don't eat salt
Rubbing the body with the hands will substitute for a bath
Bathe at midday
Don't use soap

John H. Kellogg:

Don't indulge in sex more than once per month
Women younger than 20 and men younger than 25 shouldn't have sex
Women past menopause and men older than 50 shouldn't have sex
Surgical circumcision performed before puberty will increase a girl's health
Don't squint or roll your eyes
Wear flannel neck-to-ankle underclothes year-round
Avoid developing your muscles
Bathe at 10 or 11 AM
Don't bathe when you're sweating

Table 5.3. Unverified "Whats" in *The Ministry of Healing*
(these don't appear in *Spiritual Gifts*)

Avoid eating both fruits and vegetables at any one meal
Cheese is more objectionable than butter; it is wholly unfit for food
Don't eat blood
Don't eat very hot or cold food (food should be lukewarm)
Don't allow waste vegetables or heaps of fallen leaves to remain near one's house
Don't engage in intense study immediately after eating
Don't engage in violent or excessive exercise immediately before or after eating*
Don't eat when one is excited, anxious, or hurried*
The more liquid you take with a meal, the more difficulty you'll have digesting the food*

*These items do slow digestion, but I don't consider them to be health hazards.

6

CHAPTER

Ellen G. White and Principles of Sexual Relationships

Individuals critical of Ellen White often say her views on sex reveal how unbalanced her ideas on health are. While some claim that she took a dim view of sex even within marriage, I suggest that this claim depends on a careless reading of her statements on the topic.

Considering the cultural environment in which Mrs. White lived, one might expect her to have advocated very restrictive views on sex, but she did not. Tables 5.1–5.3 indicate that her published health principles did not include any of the other reformers' strange recommendations regarding marital sexual behavior. In many of her works, however, she did write about the problems caused by "animal passions." Ron Numbers cites her counsel that Christian wives try to divert their husbands' minds "from the gratifications of lustful passions," and he notes that she regarded the husbands whose thoughts were filled with those "lustful passions" as "demons in human form" and "worse than brutes."[1] Did she, by these statements, intend to condemn even a healthy sexual relationship between spouses?

Numbers thinks that Mrs. White probably agreed with other nineteenth-century reformers who recommended sex no more often than once a month. However, he gives no evidence to support this statement; it is merely his assumption. Before reaching this conclusion, we must determine what she meant by "animal passions," "lustful passions," and husbands "worse than brutes." Was she referring to the normal sexual relationships of a loving married couple who are unselfish, kind, understanding, and passionate with each other? Or do these very negative terms sound more like a description of the insensitive behavior of a self-centered, demanding husband or even of some type of abusive behavior? What kind of relationship was she condemning?

Ellen White lived in an era when people spoke of sexual relationships with great restraint, so we can't expect her to write on this topic with the candor that is more common today. To understand what she meant, we must study carefully what she said, looking at her many statements on the subject rather than focusing on just one or two. In the following two lists, I've summarized what she wrote about good and bad marital sexual relationships.

When true love governs a husband:

- this sacred, unselfish love will control the relationship.[2]
- the young affections will be restrained until sufficient age and experience allow them to be unfettered honorably and safely.[3] [Does "unfettered" sound like once a month?]
- the husband will be careful, attentive, constant, faithful, compassionate, and full of tender love.[4]
- passion and affection, love's powerful agents, will be elevated to purity and devoted to God.[5] [Note that she didn't condemn "passion" and "affection."]
- reason will control the sexual desires and acts.[6]
- the husband will consider the result of every expression of the sexual relationship.[7]
- the sexual relationship, which God has given, will be a blessing.[8]

In contrast, here are her descriptions of the characteristics and/or results of what she calls lust and "animal passion." When these uncontrolled passions rule a husband:

- the marriage knows little of a genuine, devoted, pure love.[9]
- the husband becomes blind to consequences, not reasoning from cause to effect.[10]
- he becomes headstrong, rash, unreasonable, and defiant of all restraint.[11]
- he runs roughshod over his wife's feelings.[12]
- he controls his wife, damaging her dignity and identity because he expects her to submit to his every wish; he allows her no choice of her own.[13] [Would true love do that?]
- he treats his wife brutally.[14]
- the wife is forced to live a miserable existence, bearing one child after another.[15] [Remember, effective birth control was not available then.]
- the sexual privileges are abused.[16] [Note that they are "privileges"—something good. The bad thing is the abuse.]
- the wife's love dies out.[17]

The second list doesn't describe an unselfish, loving, sensitive relationship between spouses. Rather, it pictures a relationship that no one would approve. It isn't clear that Ellen White was saying anything about the frequency of sex; it is clear, however, that she was describing the quality of the marriage relationship.

There is another way that we can determine—perhaps with even more confidence—whether Mrs. White used the expressions *animal passions* and *lustful passions* to describe the normal sex life of loving couples or to condemn selfish, even abusive behavior. During her lifetime, some people—Adventists among them—were advocating that those who wish to be holy must refrain from sex except to have children. They said that other than for procreation, husbands and wives should live as brothers and sisters.

Ellen White's response to these ideas reveals her view of marital sex. She consistently and aggressively opposed these antisex campaigns. In fact, she said they were not from God and that such teachings "would lead to the darkest of sins and the grossest of immorality" by resulting in extramarital sexual relationships.[18]

One man had prepared a tract advocating abstinence for married couples except for procreation. He tried to get an appointment with Ellen White, hoping for her blessings on his tract. She refused to see him for a while. Eventually, however, she gave him the opportunity to present his views. When he was through, her only comment was, "Go home and be a man." He took the hint and did not publish his tract.[19]

So, Ellen White did oppose intemperate and lustful sexual relationships within marriage. But she gave balanced advice. That advice seems well summarized by the following statement:

> Jesus did not enforce celibacy upon any class of men. He came not to destroy the sacred relationship of marriage, but to exalt it and restore it to its original sanctity. He looks with pleasure upon the family relationship [sexual intercourse] where sacred and unselfish love bears sway.[20]

What About Masturbation?

Another topic relating to sexuality that Ellen White addressed has raised considerable controversy. She emphasized the dangers of "self-abuse"—a euphemism for masturbation. In 1864, she published a pamphlet entitled *Appeal to Mothers* that dealt with this topic. In 1870, James White republished almost all of it, with other material that he probably added, under the title *A Solemn Appeal.* Three sections in volume two of Ellen G. White's *Testimonies for the Church* also deal with this subject.

In the context of a dismal picture of the moral state of humanity, Ellen White portrayed long-term habits of masturbation as being common even among Seventh-day Adventist Christians. She described multiple results of these persistent habits: guilt, loss of interest in spiritual things, remorse, loss of self-respect, headache, catarrh, dizziness, nervousness, pains in the shoulder, side, back, and limbs, loss of appetite, wakefulness, tiredness, sallow countenance, absent-mindedness, sadness, impatience under restraint, and ultimately diseases of the lungs, liver, and kidneys, rheumatism, cancer, insanity, and premature death.

This long list of serious problems contrasts sharply with the common opinion of modern medicine that masturbation is harmless. Who, then, is correct about the effect of habitual self-abuse: Ellen White or modern medical opinion?

Some critics seem to think Mrs. White was saying that people who at times are overcome by their youthful hormones and masturbate are going to go insane or fall victim to the other problems on the above list. I believe this is a misunderstanding. Ellen White doesn't seem to be talking about occasional lapses. The cases she discusses with any detail involve persistent, long-term habits—even continuing through married life. She is very concerned about the life habits that people develop and the factors that can lead children down wrong paths as they make choices about life and morals.

Perhaps, however, Dr. McMahon's findings about "whats" and "whys" will also help answer our question. Ellen White's health principle—her "what"—on this issue is simple: Avoid masturbation. Don't do it. The reason for this prohibition is clear. Masturbation, pornography, and prostitution all share one feature. They distort the use of the very strong emotions that God created as part of our sexual nature. They take something that He designed to be expressed only in a tender sharing of love between two permanently united persons—a giving of joy to each other—and turn it inward, distorting it into something completely selfish, self-centered, and detached from relationships. In contrast to the "what," perhaps she didn't receive the explanation of the results of self-abuse—her "why"—by revelation. Perhaps she gleaned it from the work of other health reformers. This perspective would explain many things about how she handled this topic.

However, we shouldn't so quickly dismiss what she says. We might also take her statements as a challenge to study this topic more carefully. Modern medical science has been discovering that the mind and the body are closely tied together. The emotions that we cherish affect our physical health,[21] and our state of mind can cause many physical symptoms. Is it possible that a habitual distorted use of the powerful human sexual drive could be involved in causing health problems or at least weakening our resistance to diseases? Only research of the magnitude of the Adventist Health Study could determine whether habitual masturbation could have that result. I am not aware of such a study, so perhaps we don't know as much about this subject as we think we do. A full answer awaits further detailed medical research.

In summary, Ellen White placed a high value on the institution of marriage and the qualities of pure love, tenderness, unselfishness, and joy that it can provide. She recognized that passion and affection are powerful agents that, when devoted to God, can be safely unfettered within marriage. She was also very concerned about anything that can damage this relationship, and she expressed her concern in strong language.

Because of the way our culture has changed since her day regarding how people discuss this subject, we cannot easily assume that we completely understand what she was saying. To interpret correctly her advice on this delicate subject, we must study carefully all she says about it and place her statements in the context of her culture. In addition, more medical research must be done before we will truly know how to interpret some of what she says.

1. Numbers, 157.

2. Ellen G. White, *The Adventist Home* (Hagerstown, Md.: Review and Herald, 1952), 121.

3. Ellen G. White, *Messages to Young People* (Hagerstown, Md.: Review and Herald, 1930), 452.

4. White, *Adventist Home,* 12.

5. Ellen G. White, *Testimonies for the Church* (Nampa, Idaho: Pacific Press, 1948), 2:564.

6. Ellen G. White, *Mind, Character, and Personality* (Hagerstown, Md.: Review and Herald, 1977), 219.

7. White, *Adventist Home,* 122.

8. Ibid., 122, 124.

9. White, *Testimonies,* 2:381.

10. White, *Adventist Home,* 123.

11. Ibid., 50.

12. White, *Testimonies,* 2:381.

13. Ellen G. White, *Testimonies on Sexual Behavior, Adultery, and Divorce* (Silver Spring, Md.: The Ellen G. White Estate, 1989), 111, 112.

14. White, *Testimonies,* 2:381.

15. Ibid., 380.

16. White, *Mind, Character, and Personality,* 225.

17. White, *Testimonies on Sexual Behavior,* 112.

18. See Arthur L. White, "Ellen G. White and Marriage Relations," Parts 1 and 2, *The Ministry,* March 1969, 6–8, 26–27; and April 1969, 19–21, 23.

19. See ibid.

20. White, *Adventist Home,* 121.

21. B. L. Fredrickson, "The Value of Positive Emotions," *American Scientist,* 91:330–335.

CHAPTER 7

Conclusions

It seems evident that God has chosen to allow us each to make our own decisions about our belief system. He does not hinder us from making a free choice, though our choices have consequences for good or ill. As Christians, as Adventists, we should also refrain from attempting to control the decisions others make. So, we shouldn't object to people holding opinions different from our own on these issues of the nature of inspiration.

However, when people challenge the divine inspiration and reliability of either the Bible or the writings of Ellen G. White, then we have a right to expect that they have based their challenges on a high-quality examination of the evidence, with the very best approach to research design. When instead the challengers have based their research on a very inadequate research design and faulty logic, such as we find in the publications by Rea, Butler, and Numbers, then we have a right to be skeptical of their conclusions.

Our research has revealed serious weaknesses in the arguments of these critics of Mrs. White. Their claims that her writings can be explained as originating from strictly human sources do not stand up to critical evaluation. Dr. Don McMahon's research reveals a dramatic difference in quality between Mrs. White's health principles and those advocated by other health reformers in the 1800s. Modern medical science has verified a high percentage of her health principles (the "whats"), while the sources from which she supposedly copied had a low percentage of health principles that have been verified. This difference indicates that Mrs. White had health information that could not have come from any human source available anywhere at the time she lived and wrote. The charge that she copied her health principles from other health reformers does not even come close to being realistic. At least in the area of health, our research has provided evidence that demands an extrabiblical, extrahuman source of information to account for the accuracy of her health principles.

Yet it is clear that many of the physiological explanations (the "whys") that she gave were consistent with the limited medical knowledge of her time and do not fit the prevailing model of divine inspiration. It appears that God has told us what we need to know to live safely, but He hasn't provided all the explanations as to the reasons behind these "whats." If we trust the medical and spiritual principles He has given us, our lives and spiritual experience will benefit. But if we expect to understand all the "whys" before we do the "whats," we may never find a basis for trusting Him. We can improve in our understanding of God-given principles as we study more; apparently, He has left us to figure out the explanations by using the brains He gave us. As we seek these explanations, we'll need to humbly trust His revealed will.

In science, the constant give and take of mutual constructive criticism encourages a degree of objectivity and improved accuracy. Likewise, in our analysis of the prophetic gift, a constructive give and take will improve our confidence in our conclusions. So, we welcome critical analysis of our work and will respond by correcting any mistakes we may have made or in pointing out the errors of our critics, whichever a careful study indicates is needed.

Health Principles and Legalism

So, the evidence presented in this book indicates that God gave us the health principles contained in the writings of Ellen G. White. Why did He bother to give them to us? And why should we take the trouble to live by them? Isn't it legalistic to try to earn heavenly merit by following lifestyle rules?

God loves us so much that He not only died to assure our salvation, but He also took the trouble to give us insights into healthful, happy living. There is nothing legalistic about that. We don't earn salvation points by living healthy lives. But we do give glory to God by becoming living demonstrations of the benefits of trusting Him and following His advice. How could we slap the face of our very best Friend in the whole universe and by our actions say to Him, "We don't care what You say; we'll live as we please"?

Our study has another important implication. Ellen White wrote much about preparation for the return of Jesus to this earth and preparation for a confident dependence on God through the turmoil that will precede His return. If God inspired her health writings, does it seem likely that He would leave her to randomly copy false material in other subjects important to our salvation and our relationship to Him?

Mrs. White stated repeatedly that her role was to uplift Jesus and to encourage us to trust the Bible and make it the foundation of our faith. She also, through her writings, gave us a beautiful picture of a loving God who seeks us and who offers us His grace for our every spiritual need. By faith we accept forgiveness, salvation, guidance, and strength for Christian growth. These are all gifts from God. We do not deserve them, but God gives them freely by His grace. Whether or not we benefit by them is up to us. We also choose whether we will listen to and believe God's communication to us through His messengers, which, in His kindness and love, He has given to protect us from being deceived by the enemy of us all.

Appendix
Prophets and Kings and *Night Scenes in the Bible*

Walter Rea's book *The White Lie* contains exhibits that compare material from Ellen White's books to that of her sources. In making his exhibits, Rea extracted only the parallel materials from the various books. Without the larger context, readers don't get an accurate sense of how much—or how little—material Mrs. White was using from her sources.

The exhibit that follows consists of most of two chapters from Ellen G. White's *Prophets and Kings* and the parallel section of Daniel March's *Night Scenes in the Bible.* This allows the reader to gain a more accurate picture of how much similarity or dissimilarity there actually is between the two books—in other words, of how "dependent" Mrs. White was on March's book.

Underlined portions of the two books are essentially the same. Some other material may have similar themes, but the wording differs. The examples given here are the ones Walter Rea used. Mrs. White may also have used other sources for the passage reproduced; that's outside the purview of this study.

The Story of

PROPHETS

and

KINGS

As Illustrated in the Captivity and Restoration of Israel

by ELLEN G. WHITE

Author of "Patriarchs and Prophets," "The Acts of the Apostles," "The Desire of Ages," and "The Great Controversy"

PACIFIC PRESS® PUBLISHING ASSOCIATION
Nampa, Idaho
Oshawa, Ontario, Canada

11

Carmel

STANDING before Ahab, Elijah demanded that all Israel be assembled to meet him and the prophets of Baal and Ashtoreth on Mount Carmel. "Send," he commanded, "and gather to me all Israel unto Mount Carmel, and the prophets of Baal four hundred and fifty, and the prophets of the groves four hundred, which eat at Jezebel's table."

The command was issued by one who seemed to stand in the very presence of Jehovah; and Ahab obeyed at once, as if the prophet were monarch, and the king a subject. Swift messengers were sent throughout the kingdom with the summons to meet Elijah and the prophets of Baal and Ashtoreth. In every town and village the people prepared to assemble at the appointed time. As they journeyed toward the place, the hearts of many were filled with strange forebodings. Something unusual was about to happen; else why this summons to gather at Carmel? What

This chapter is based on 1 Kings 18:19-40.

new calamity was about to fall upon the people and the land?

Before the drought, Mount Carmel had been a place of beauty, its streams fed from never-failing springs, and its fertile slopes covered with fair flowers and flourishing groves. But now its beauty languished under a withering curse. The altars erected to the worship of Baal and Ashtoreth stood now in leafless groves. On the summit of one of the highest ridges, in sharp contrast with these was the broken-down altar of Jehovah.

Carmel overlooked a wide expanse of country; its heights were visible from many parts of the kingdom of Israel. At the foot of the mount there were vantage points from which could be seen much of what took place above. God had been signally dishonored by the idolatrous worship carried on under cover of its wooded slopes; and Elijah chose this elevation as the most conspicuous place for the display of God's power and for the vindication of the honor of His name.

Early on the morning of the day appointed, the hosts of apostate Israel, in eager expectancy, gather near the top of the mountain. Jezebel's prophets march up in imposing array. In regal pomp the king appears and takes his position at the head of the priests, and the idolaters shout his welcome. But there is apprehension in the hearts of the priests as they remember that at the word of the prophet the land of Israel for three years and a half has been destitute of dew and rain. Some fearful crisis is at hand, they feel sure. The gods in whom they have trusted have been unable to prove Elijah a false prophet. To their frantic cries, their prayers, their tears, their humiliation, their revolting ceremonies, their costly and ceaseless sacrifices, the objects of their worship have been strangely indifferent.

Facing King Ahab and the false prophets, and surrounded by the assembled hosts of Israel, Elijah stands, the only one who has appeared to vindicate the honor of Jehovah. He whom the whole kingdom has charged with its weight of woe is now before them, apparently defenseless in the presence of the monarch of Israel, the prophets of Baal, the men of war, and the surrounding thousands. But Elijah is not alone. Above and around him are the protecting hosts of heaven, angels that excel in strength.

Unashamed, unterrified, the prophet stands before the multitude, fully aware of his commission to execute the divine command. His countenance is lighted with an awful solemnity. In anxious expectancy the people wait for him to speak. Looking first upon the broken-down altar of Jehovah, and then upon the multitude, Elijah cries out in clear, trumpetlike tones, "How long halt ye between two opinions? if the Lord be God, follow Him: but if Baal, then follow him."

The people answer him not a word. Not one in that vast assembly dare reveal loyalty to Jehovah. Like a dark cloud, deception and blindness had overspread Israel. Not all at once had this fatal apostasy closed about them, but gradually, as from time to time they had failed to heed the words of warning and reproof that the Lord sent them. Each departure from rightdoing, each refusal to repent, had deepened their guilt and driven them farther from Heaven. And now, in this crisis, they persisted in refusing to take their stand for God.

The Lord abhors indifference and disloyalty in a time of crisis in His work. The whole universe is watching with inexpressible interest the closing scenes of the great controversy between good and evil. The people of God are nearing the borders of the eternal world; what can be of more importance to them than that they be loyal to the God of heaven? All through the ages, God has had moral heroes, and He has them now—those who, like Joseph and Elijah and Daniel, are not ashamed to acknowledge themselves His peculiar people. His special blessing accompanies the labors of men of action, men who will not be swerved from the straight line of duty, but who with divine energy will inquire, "Who is on the Lord's side?" (Exodus 32:26), men who will not stop merely with the inquiry, but who will demand that those who choose to identify themselves with the people of God shall step forward and reveal unmistakably their allegiance to the King of kings and Lord of lords. Such men make their wills and plans subordinate to the law of God. For love of Him they count not their lives dear unto themselves. Their work is to catch the light from the Word and let it shine forth to the world in clear, steady rays. Fidelity to God is their motto.

While Israel on Carmel doubt and hesitate, the voice of Elijah again breaks the silence: "I, even I only, remain a prophet of the Lord; but Baal's prophets are four hundred and fifty men. Let them therefore give us two bullocks; and let them choose one bullock for themselves, and cut it in pieces, and lay it on wood, and put no fire under: and I will dress the other bullock, and lay it on wood, and put no fire under: and call ye on the name of your gods, and

I will call on the name of the Lord: and the God that answereth by fire, let him be God."

The proposal of Elijah is so reasonable that the people cannot well evade it, so they find courage to answer, "It is well spoken." The prophets of Baal dare not lift their voices in dissent; and, addressing them, Elijah directs, "Choose you one bullock for yourselves, and dress it first; for ye are many; and call on the name of your gods, but put no fire under."

Outwardly bold and defiant, but with terror in their guilty hearts, the false priests prepare their altar, laying on the wood and the victim; and then they begin their incantations. Their shrill cries echo and re-echo through the forests and the surrounding heights, as they call on the name of their god, saying, "O Baal, hear us." The priests gather about their altar, and with leaping and writhing and screaming, with tearing of hair and cutting of flesh, they beseech their god to help them.

The morning passes, noon comes, and yet there is no evidence that Baal hears the cries of his deluded followers. There is no voice, no reply to their frantic prayers. The sacrifice remains unconsumed.

As they continue their frenzied devotions, the crafty priests are continually trying to devise some means by which they may kindle a fire upon the altar and lead the people to believe that the fire has come direct from Baal. But Elijah watches every movement; and the priests, hoping against hope for some opportunity to deceive, continue to carry on their senseless ceremonies.

"It came to pass at noon, that Elijah mocked them, and

said, Cry aloud: for he is a god; either he is talking, or he is pursuing, or he is in a journey, or peradventure he sleepeth, and must be awaked. And they cried aloud, and cut themselves after their manner with knives and lancets, till the blood gushed out upon them. And it came to pass, when midday was past, and they prophesied until the time of the offering of the evening sacrifice, that there was neither voice, nor any to answer, nor any that regarded."

Gladly would Satan have come to the help of those whom he had deceived, and who were devoted to his service. Gladly would he have sent the lightning to kindle their sacrifice. But Jehovah has set Satan's bounds, restrained his power, and not all the enemy's devices can convey one spark to Baal's altar.

At last, their voices hoarse with shouting, their garments stained with blood from self-inflicted wounds, the priests become desperate. With unabated frenzy they now mingle with their pleading terrible cursings of their sun-god, and Elijah continues to watch intently; for he knows that if by any device the priests should succeed in kindling their altar fire, he would instantly be torn in pieces.

Evening draws on. The prophets of Baal are weary, faint, confused. One suggests one thing, and another something else, until finally they cease their efforts. Their shrieks and curses no longer resound over Carmel. In despair they retire from the contest.

All day long the people have witnessed the demonstrations of the baffled priests. They have beheld their wild leaping round the altar, as if they would grasp the burning rays of the sun to serve their purpose. They have looked with horror on the frightful, self-inflicted mutilations of the priests, and have had opportunity to reflect on the follies of idol worship. Many in the throng are weary of the exhibitions of demonism, and they now await with deepest interest the movements of Elijah.

It is the hour of the evening sacrifice, and Elijah bids the people, "Come near unto me." As they tremblingly draw near, he turns to the broken-down altar where once men worshiped the God of heaven, and repairs it. To him this heap of ruins is more precious than all the magnificent altars of heathendom.

In the reconstruction of this ancient altar, Elijah revealed his respect for the covenant that the Lord made with Israel when they crossed the Jordan into the Promised Land. Choosing "twelve stones, according to the number of the tribes of the sons of Jacob, . . . he built an altar in the name of the Lord."

The disappointed priests of Baal, exhausted by their vain efforts, wait to see what Elijah will do. They hate the prophet for proposing a test that has exposed the weakness and inefficiency of their gods; yet they fear his power. The people, fearful also, and almost breathless with expectancy, watch while Elijah continues his preparations. The calm demeanor of the prophet stands out in sharp contrast with the fanatical, senseless frenzy of the followers of Baal.

The altar completed, the prophet makes a trench about it, and, having put the wood in order and prepared the bullock, he lays the victim on the altar and commands the people to flood the sacrifice and the altar with water. "Fill four barrels," he directed, "and pour it on the burnt sacrifice, and on the wood. And he said, Do it the second time. And they did it the second time. And he said, Do it the third time. And they did it the third time. And the water ran round about the altar; and he filled the trench also with water."

Reminding the people of the long-continued apostasy that has awakened the wrath of Jehovah, Elijah calls upon them to humble their hearts and turn to the God of their fathers, that the curse upon the land of Israel may be removed. Then, bowing reverently before the unseen God, he raises his hands toward heaven and offers a simple prayer. Baal's priests have screamed and foamed and leaped, from early morning until late in the afternoon; but as Elijah prays, no senseless shrieks resound over Carmel's height. He prays as if he knows Jehovah is there, a witness to the scene, a listener to his appeal. The prophets of Baal have prayed wildly, incoherently. Elijah prays simply and fervently, asking God to show His superiority over Baal, that Israel may be led to turn to Him.

"Lord God of Abraham, Isaac, and of Israel," the prophet pleads, "let it be known this day that Thou art God in Israel, and that I am Thy servant, and that I have done all these things at Thy word. Hear me, O Lord, hear me, that this people may know that Thou art the Lord God, and that Thou hast turned their heart back again."

A silence, oppressive in its solemnity, rests upon all. The priests of Baal tremble with terror. Conscious of their guilt, they look for swift retribution.

No sooner is the prayer of Elijah ended than flames of

fire, like brilliant flashes of lightning, descend from heaven upon the upreared altar, consuming the sacrifice, licking up the water in the trench, and consuming even the stones of the altar. The brilliancy of the blaze illumines the mountain and dazzles the eyes of the multitude. In the valleys below, where many are watching in anxious suspense the movements of those above, the descent of fire is clearly seen, and all are amazed at the sight. It resembles the pillar of fire which at the Red Sea separated the children of Israel from the Egyptian host.

The people on the mount prostrate themselves in awe before the unseen God. They dare not continue to look upon the Heaven-sent fire. They fear that they themselves will be consumed; and, convicted of their duty to acknowledge the God of Elijah as the God of their fathers, to whom they owe allegiance, they cry out together as with one voice, "The Lord, He is the God; the Lord, He is the God." With startling distinctness the cry resounds over the mountain and echoes in the plain below. At last Israel is aroused, undeceived, penitent. At last the people see how greatly they have dishonored God. The character of Baal worship, in contrast with the reasonable service required by the true God, stands fully revealed. The people recognize God's justice and mercy in withholding the dew and the rain until they have been brought to confess His name. They are ready now to admit that the God of Elijah is above every idol.

The priests of Baal witness with consternation the wonderful revelation of Jehovah's power. Yet even in their discomfiture and in the presence of divine glory, they refuse to repent of their evil-doing. They would still remain the prophets of Baal. Thus they showed themselves ripe for destruction. That repentant Israel may be protected from the allurements of those who have taught them to worship Baal, Elijah is directed by the Lord to destroy these false teachers. The anger of the people has already been aroused against the leaders in transgression; and when Elijah gives the command, "Take the prophets of Baal; let not one of them escape," they are ready to obey. They seize the priests, and take them to the brook Kishon, and there, before the close of the day that marked the beginning of decided reform, the ministers of Baal are slain. Not one is permitted to live.

12

From Jezreel to Horeb

WITH the slaying of the prophets of Baal, the way was opened for carrying forward a mighty spiritual reformation among the ten tribes of the northern kingdom. Elijah had set before the people their apostasy; he had called upon them to humble their hearts and turn to the Lord. The judgments of Heaven had been executed; the people had confessed their sins, and had acknowledged the God of their fathers as the living God; and now the curse of Heaven was to be withdrawn, and the temporal blessings of life renewed. The land was to be refreshed with rain. "Get thee up, eat and drink," Elijah said to Ahab; "for there is a sound of abundance of rain." Then the prophet went to the top of the mount to pray.

It was not because of any outward evidence that the showers were about to fall, that Elijah could so confidently bid Ahab prepare for rain. The prophet saw no clouds in the heavens; he heard no thunder. He simply spoke the

This chapter is based on 1 Kings 18:41-46; 19:1-8.

word that the Spirit of the Lord had moved him to speak in response to his own strong faith. Throughout the day he had unflinchingly performed the will of God and had revealed his implicit confidence in the prophecies of God's word; and now, having done all that was in his power to do, he knew that Heaven would freely bestow the blessings foretold. The same God who had sent the drought had promised an abundance of rain as the reward of rightdoing; and now Elijah waited for the promised outpouring. In an attitude of humility, "his face between his knees," he interceded with God in behalf of penitent Israel.

Again and again Elijah sent his servant to a point overlooking the Mediterranean, to learn whether there were any visible token that God had heard his prayer. Each time the servant returned with the word, "There is nothing." The prophet did not become impatient or lose faith, but continued his earnest pleading. Six times the servant returned with the word that there was no sign of rain in the brassy heavens. Undaunted, Elijah sent him forth once more; and this time the servant returned with the word, "Behold, there ariseth a little cloud out of the sea, like a man's hand."

This was enough. Elijah did not wait for the heavens to gather blackness. In that small cloud he beheld by faith an abundance of rain; and he acted in harmony with his faith, sending his servant quickly to Ahab with the message, "Prepare thy chariot, and get thee down, that the rain stop thee not."

It was because Elijah was a man of large faith that God could use him in this grave crisis in the history of Israel.

As he prayed, his faith reached out and grasped the promises of Heaven, and he persevered in prayer until his petitions were answered. He did not wait for the full evidence that God had heard him, but was willing to venture all on the slightest token of divine favor. And yet what he was enabled to do under God, all may do in their sphere of activity in God's service; for of the prophet from the mountains of Gilead it is written: "Elias was a man subject to like passions as we are, and he prayed earnestly that it might not rain: and it rained not on the earth by the space of three years and six months." James 5:17.

Faith such as this is needed in the world today—faith that will lay hold on the promises of God's word and refuse to let go until Heaven hears. Faith such as this connects us closely with Heaven, and brings us strength for coping with the powers of darkness. Through faith God's children have "subdued kingdoms, wrought righteousness, obtained promises, stopped the mouths of lions, quenched the violence of fire, escaped the edge of the sword, out of weakness were made strong, waxed valiant in fight, turned to flight the armies of the aliens." Hebrews 11:33, 34. And through faith we today are to reach the heights of God's purpose for us. "If thou canst believe, all things are possible to him that believeth." Mark 9:23.

Faith is an essential element of prevailing prayer. "He that cometh to God must believe that He is, and that He is a rewarder of them that diligently seek Him." "If we ask anything according to His will, He heareth us: and if we know that He hear us, whatsoever we ask, we know that we have the petitions that we desired of Him." Hebrews 11:6; 1 John 5:14, 15. With the persevering faith of Jacob, with the unyielding persistence of Elijah, we may present our petitions to the Father, claiming all that He has promised. The honor of His throne is staked for the fulfillment of His word.

The shades of night were gathering about Mount Carmel as Ahab prepared for the descent. "It came to pass in the meanwhile, that the heaven was black with clouds and wind, and there was a great rain. And Ahab rode, and went to Jezreel." As he journeyed toward the royal city through the darkness and the blinding rain, Ahab was unable to see his way before him. Elijah, who, as the prophet of God, had that day humiliated Ahab before his subjects and slain his idolatrous priests, still acknowledged him as Israel's king; and now, as an act of homage, and strengthened by the power of God, he ran before the royal chariot, guiding the king to the entrance of the city.

In this gracious act of God's messenger shown to a wicked king is a lesson for all who claim to be servants of God, but who are exalted in their own estimation. There are those who feel above performing duties that to them appear menial. They hesitate to perform even needful service, fearing that they will be found doing the work of a servant. These have much to learn from the example of Elijah. By his word the treasures of heaven had been for three years withheld from the earth; he had been signally honored of God as, in answer to his prayer on Carmel, fire had flashed from heaven and consumed the sacrifice; his hand had executed the judgment of God in slaying the idolatrous prophets; his petition for rain had been granted. And yet, after the signal triumphs with which God had been pleased to honor his public ministry, he was willing to perform the service of a menial.

At the gate of Jezreel, Elijah and Ahab separated. The prophet, choosing to remain outside the walls, wrapped himself in his mantle, and lay down upon the bare earth to sleep. The king, passing within, soon reached the shelter of his palace and there related to his wife the wonderful events of the day and the marvelous revelation of divine power that had proved to Israel that Jehovah is the true God and Elijah His chosen messenger. As Ahab told the queen of the slaying of the idolatrous prophets, Jezebel, hardened and impenitent, became infuriated. She refused to recognize in the events on Carmel the overruling providence of God, and, still defiant, she boldly declared that Elijah should die.

That night a messenger aroused the weary prophet and delivered to him the word of Jezebel: "So let the gods do to me, and more also, if I make not thy life as the life of one of them by tomorrow about this time."

It would seem that after showing courage so undaunted, after triumphing so completely over king and priests and people, Elijah could never afterward have given way to despondency nor been awed into timidity. But he who had been blessed with so many evidences of God's loving care was not above the frailties of mankind, and in this dark hour his faith and courage forsook him. Bewildered, he started from his slumber. The rain was pouring from the heavens, and darkness was on every side. Forgetting that three years before, God had directed his course to a place of refuge from the hatred of Jezebel and the search of Ahab, the prophet now fled for his life. Reaching Beersheba, he "left his servant there. But he himself went a day's journey into the wilderness."

Elijah should not have fled from his post of duty. He should have met the threat of Jezebel with an appeal for protection to the One who had commissioned him to vindicate the honor of Jehovah. He should have told the messenger that the God in whom he trusted would protect him against the hatred of the queen. Only a few hours had passed since he had witnessed a wonderful manifestation of divine power, and this should have given him assurance that he would not now be forsaken. Had he remained where he was, had he made God his refuge and strength, standing steadfast for the truth, he would have been shielded from harm. The Lord would have given him another signal victory by sending His judgments on Jezebel; and the impression made on the king and the people would have wrought a great reformation.

Elijah had expected much from the miracle wrought on Carmel. He had hoped that after this display of God's power, Jezebel would no longer have influence over the mind of Ahab, and that there would be a speedy reform throughout Israel. All day on Carmel's height he had toiled without food. Yet when he guided the chariot of Ahab to the gate of Jezreel, his courage was strong, despite the physical strain under which he had labored.

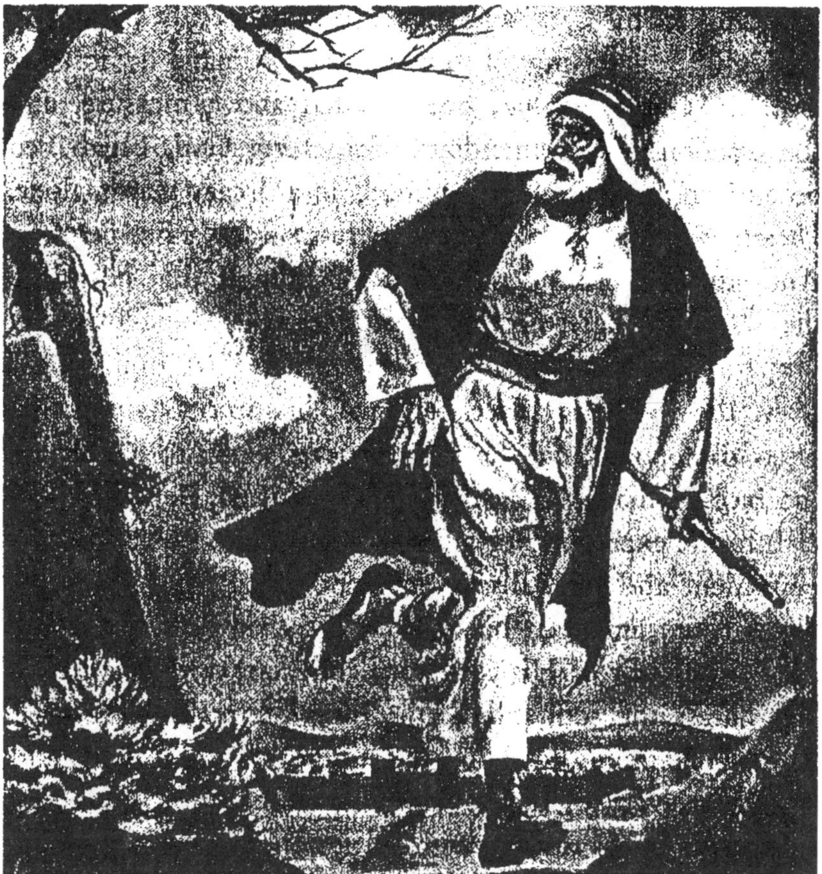

DON HUTH, ARTIST © P. P. P. A.

Fearful of Queen Jezebel's threat against his life, Elijah forgot his duty to God by running away in search of a place of refuge.

But a reaction such as frequently follows high faith and glorious success was pressing upon Elijah. He feared that the reformation begun on Carmel might not be lasting; and depression seized him. He had been exalted to Pisgah's top; now he was in the valley. While under the inspiration of the Almighty, he had stood the severest trial of faith; but in this time of discouragement, with Jezebel's threat

6—P.K.

sounding in his ears, and Satan still apparently prevailing through the plotting of this wicked woman, he lost his hold on God. He had been exalted above measure, and the reaction was tremendous. Forgetting God, Elijah fled on and on, until he found himself in a dreary waste, alone. Utterly wearied, he sat down to rest under a juniper tree. And sitting there, he requested for himself that he might die. "It is enough; now, O Lord," he said, "take away my life; for I am not better than my fathers." A fugitive, far from the dwelling places of men, his spirits crushed by bitter disappointment, he desired never again to look upon the face of man. At last, utterly exhausted, he fell asleep.

Into the experience of all there come times of keen disappointment and utter discouragement—days when sorrow is the portion, and it is hard to believe that God is still the kind benefactor of His earthborn children; days when troubles harass the soul, till death seems preferable to life. It is then that many lose their hold on God and are brought into the slavery of doubt, the bondage of unbelief. Could we at such times discern with spiritual insight the meaning of God's providences we should see angels seeking to save us from ourselves, striving to plant our feet upon a foundation more firm than the everlasting hills, and new faith, new life, would spring into being.

The faithful Job, in the day of his affliction and darkness, declared:

> "Let the day perish wherein I was born."
> "O that my grief were throughly weighed,
> And my calamity laid in the balances together!"

"O that I might have my request;
And that God would grant me the thing that I long for!
Even that it would please God to destroy me;
That He would let loose His hand, and cut me off!
Then should I yet have comfort."

"I will not refrain my mouth;
I will speak in the anguish of my spirit;
I will complain in the bitterness of my soul."

"My soul chooseth . . . death rather than my life.
I loathe it;
I would not live alway:
Let me alone;
For my days are vanity."
Job 3:3; 6:2, 8-10; 7:11, 15, 16.

But though weary of life, Job was not allowed to die. To him were pointed out the possibilities of the future, and there was given him the message of hope:

"Thou shalt be steadfast, and shalt not fear:
Because thou shalt forget thy misery,
And remember it as waters that pass away:
And thine age shall be clearer than the noonday;
Thou shalt shine forth, thou shalt be as the morning.
And thou shalt be secure,
Because there is hope. . . .
Thou shalt lie down,
And none shall make thee afraid;
Yea, many shall make suit unto thee.
But the eyes of the wicked shall fail,
And they shall not escape,
And their hope shall be as the giving up of the ghost."
Job 11:15-20.

From the depths of discouragement and despondency Job rose to the heights of implicit trust in the mercy and the saving power of God. Triumphantly he declared:

NIGHT SCENES

IN THE

BIBLE.

BY

REV. DANIEL MARCH, D.D

AUTHOR OF "WALKS AND HOMES OF JESUS."

ZEIGLER & McCURDY,
PHILADELPHIA, PA.; CINCINNATI, OHIO;
CHICAGO, ILL.; ST. LOUIS, MO.
SPRINGFIELD, MASS.
1870.

in the third year, saying, Go show thyself unto Ahab; and I will send rain upon the earth."

With him, to receive the word of the Lord was to obey. He had been outlawed and hated and hunted down by all the power of the king for three years, and the whole nation had been put under oath that the prophet could be nowhere found. And now, unbidden by the king, without explanation or apology, Elijah comes forth from his seclusion. Himself assuming to be the monarch, he sends a messenger to say, "Behold! Elijah is here." If Ahab wants to see him, he can come. The prophet will not go to him. And when the king makes haste to come, Elijah demands a solemn convocation of all Israel and of the prophets of Baal at Carmel. For three years Ahab had been sending spies through all the land of Israel and the neighboring kingdoms to find Elijah, that he might put him to death; and now that he meets him face to face the passionate king is so awed and unmanned by the presence of the prophet that he only obeys at once when commanded, as if Elijah were king and Ahab were the subject and slave.

Swift couriers are sent throughout all the kingdom with the summons, and every village and family gladly sends its representative to the great assembly. All who have strength for the journey are in haste to answer the call of Elijah and the word of the king. The place of gathering was already sacred, and it was in sight of a large portion of the kingdom. The highways and the footpaths among the hills are alive with people moving in one direction. Clouds of dust arise and darken the sultry air, as the long lines of the gathering multitude stream across the great plain of Jezreel toward the wooded heights of Carmel. Jezebel's eight hundred and fifty prophets of Baal and Astarte march out in one body from their great temple, like a regiment of soldiers moving to battle, with banners flying and flushed with the hope of victory. At last a blaze of bright spears and burnished shields flashes across the plain, and the dust-cloud rolls as if caught in a whirlwind where the chariot of Ahab passes swiftly, with panting footmen running before and galloping horsemen riding behind. And when the sun goes down, an innumerable multitude are encamped on the eastern slope of the wooded mountain, waiting some great and awful decision on the morrow.

When the day is fully come, and the morning sun struggles through the murky air on the east, a sudden murmur runs through the great encampment—there is a flowing in of the straggling multitude toward one central position—for, behold! Elijah, with awful look and shaggy mantle, is there. The one man on whom a whole kingdom had laid the weight of its desolation and its agony, stands before them unterrified, defenceless, alone!

On the highest ridge of the mountain, where the altar of Jehovah had once stood and had been thrown down, in full view of the great plain and the temple

14

of Baal at Jezreel, and the high places of idolatrous worship around Samaria, the prophet comes forth and takes his stand. All down the wooded slope of the mountain, under the shade of oaks and olive trees, in orchards and gardens are gathered the thousands of the people, waiting with breathless awe and expectation to catch the first word from the lips of the man who ever spoke as in the presence of the Lord of hosts. Nearer, and hemmed in by the multitude around a fountain of water which flows to this day, are the false prophets and their patron king.

In the open light of day, under the broad canopy of heaven, with eager thousands to see and to hear, Elijah cries aloud, "How long halt ye between two opinions? If Jehovah be God, follow him. but if Baal, then follow him." But there is not one in all the multitude that dares to utter an approving word or give a sign of assent to a proposition so plain. Again the lonely prophet of Jehovah speaks, and challenges the priests of Baal to join with him in rearing two altars and laying on the sacrifice, and each calling upon their own object of worship, and the God that answereth by fire let him be God. And now the people are emboldened to answer, "The word is good."

The priests of Baal, cannot escape the trial. They rear their own altar, lay on the wood and the victim, and then they begin to chant and howl, in the wild orgies of idolatrous worship, until the whole forest of Carmel resounds with their cries, "Oh Baal, hear us?"

They surround their altar like a legion of demons, with a whirling and giddy dance, leaping up and down, tossing and tearing their many-colored and fantastic robes, growing more rapid and furious in their motions and more wild and frantic in their cries as the slow hours of the morning pass on and the sultry noon comes and there is no voice nor any that answers. It is past midday, and still, hoping to gain time and find some device or sleight of hand by which the fire can be kindled, they continue their cries, cutting their flesh, leaping over the altar, staining their faces and their garments with their blood, howling and foaming with frantic excitement, making the whole mountain resound with the demoniac chorus of eight hundred hoarse and screaming voices, mingling curses with their prayers to their pitiless sun-god for the answer of fire, and still it does not come.

All the while Elijah stands alone, waiting and knowing full well that if by any deceit or cunning they should kindle the altar the people will join with them in tearing him in pieces on the spot. He even provokes and goads them on, telling them to call louder that their god may be awaked. But all in vain for the frantic and fainting priests of Baal. There is none to answer nor any that regards The people are weary of the vain repetitions and terrible demonism of idolatry.

And now it is time for Elijah to take his turn. Again he lifts up his voice, and the people crowd to hear. The maddened priests of Baal, reeking with blood, exhausted with their own frenzy, sink in silence on the ground. With calm and solemn deportment, Elijah rebuilds the altar of Jehovah with twelve stones, according to the number of the tribes of Israel, lays on the wood and the victim for the sacrifice, and then causes it to be flooded with water three times over. And then, at the hour of the evening sacrifice, the prophet stands forth alone and calls upon the name of Jehovah, the everlasting God. The great multitude are pale and breathless with awful expectation while he speaks. His calm and simple prayer and his peaceful deportment are more impressive than the foaming fury and the wild cries of a thousand priests of Baal.

No sooner has he spoken than the rushing flame descends from the clear heavens like the lightning's flash, and the very stones of the altar are burnt up with the devouring fire. The sudden blaze blinds the eyes of the multitude and illumines the whole slope of the mountain with a light above the brightness of the sun. The people watching afar off, on the house-tops in Jezreel and Samaria, and on the hills of Ephraim and Galilee, are startled at the sight. It seems to them as if the pillar of fire that led their fathers in the desert had descended upon Carmel. The multitude on the mountain fall on their faces to the ground, unable to look upon the great light, and they cry with one voice, "Jehovah is God! Jehovah is God!" In the wild excitement of the moment they rush upon the false prophets with one accord, drag them down to the river Kishon, and there Elijah himself, the terrible and strong servant of Jehovah, slays them with his own hand, according as it had been commanded in the law of Moses. The ancient Kishon ran blood all the way to the sea, and the slain worshipers of Baal were piled in heaps higher than all the altars they had reared to their false god.

And now that the people have confessed their father's God and the false prophets are slain, it is time for the rain to come and for the parched earth to revive again with returning life. Elijah goes up from the terrible sacrifice to the top of the mount in such a mood that he can still pray. He continues his supplications until his servant has come six times from his outlook over the sea to say that there was nothing in sight but the glassy, heaving wave and the coppery, cloudless sky where the sun had gone down. At the seventh time, he can only say that there is a handful of mist hanging on the horizon, as if a sea-bird had shaken the spray from her wing in the air. But it is enough. Elijah, to whom all signs and aspects of the clouds and sky have been familiar from his youth, can already hear the sound of the coming tempest.

And now the prophet warns Ahab to hasten down to the plain and mount his chariot and drive swiftly, lest the blinding storm and the swollen stream of the Kishon make it impossible for him to reach Jezreel that night. And then, after all the terrible excitement and exhausting toil of that day, this strange and strong man, Elijah, girt his rough mantle close about his loins, took his stand before the chariot of the king, and ran ll the way, fifteen miles, across the plain, through darkness and wind and mire and a deluge of rain, before the flying horses of the king, to the gate of the city, and then, like an Arab of modern times, he would not go in, but stayed outside the walls and cast himself upon the bare earth, in the midst of the storm, for his night's repose. The prophet had put the king to shame before his people at Carmel, and he ran before his chariot as an act of homage to show that he still acknowledged him as his sovereign. He who could call down fire from heaven, and bring the clouds and the rain, was still willing to perform the menial service of running in the rain and darkness before the chariot of his king.

We should suppose that no threat or violence could terrify such a man in the least. After having faced the king, the false prophets and the people, and completely triumphed over them all in a contest of life and death, we should suppose that he would be just the man to awe the furious queen in her own palace and rebuild the altar of Jehovah in the capital of the kingdom.

But no. That very night, in the midst of the darkness and the storm, a messenger came out from the city gate, roused the weary prophet from his first slumber, and shouted into his ear the oath of Jezebel, sworn by all the gods of Tyre and Sidon, that before another sun had set she would do unto him as he had done unto the prophets of Baal. We wait to hear in what terms this iron-hearted saint and hero will hurl back his defiance upon the queen in the name of the Lord of hosts.

But instead of that he rises like one terrified by a dream and not yet fully awake. Wet, cold, begrimed with mud and his garments still dabbled with gore, he springs to his feet, looks this way and that for a moment and then flees for his life. Over the hills of Samaria and the mountains of Ephraim, up and down the stony paths of Bethel and Gibeon, along the bed of the wild valleys west of Jerusalem and Bethlehem, and then out upon the plain of Sharon to Beersheba, he hurries like some conscience-smitten murderer who sees the avenger of blood behind him in every shadow.

Nor does he dare to rest, even in the farthest town of the kingdom of Judah. Leaving his only attendant behind him, without guide or provision for the way, he starts out in the early morning upon the waste and lifeless desert. All day long he toils over the broken hills and barren plains of yellow sand and bare earth. The dead uniformity of desolation stretches in every direction to the horizon. No living thing moves upon the earth or flies in the hot and glimmering air. Now and then a suffocating blast sweeps over the horrible wilderness, and the shining sand rises and whirls in waves and columns of fire. And still he presses silently on till the sun goes down and the stars come out in the sky. Then, finding a low, solitary bush of desert-broom, he casts himself beneath it, weary, hungry, and in such complete despair that he would rather die than live.

Such is the reaction which not unfrequently follows the most daring effort and the most dazzling success. Such is the despondency that sometimes presses hard upon the most sublime and heroic faith in the purest and noblest minds.

Peter drew his sword against a multitude in defence of his Master, and the next hour he was frightened out of all faith and courage by the scornful finger of a little maid.

Paul was caught up to the third heaven in visions of glory and Paradise, and he heard words of wondrous and ineffable meaning, such as cannot be spoken to ears of flesh and blood; and then, soon after, the same favored apostle was praying with thrice-repeated and beseeching supplication to be delivered from some common and petty annoyance, such as tries the temper and disturbs the peace of every one of us every day of life.

The Christian Pilgrim, in Bunyan's truthful and ingenious allegory, lodged in the palace Beautiful and slept in the chamber called Peace. In the morning he saw the Delectable Mountains and Immanuel's land from the housetop. He started forth upon his journey harnessed from head to foot in armor of proof. And yet he had gone but a little way before "he began to be afraid, and to cast in his mind whether to go back or to press on." The beautiful vision and the fair prospect of the morning were followed by the valley of Humiliation and the most desperate and agonizing conflict with Apollyon.

The young disciple of Christ rejoices in the freshness of his first love, and he feels that he would gladly go to the ends of the earth for his new Master. Frank and fearless in his faith and zeal, he is ready to speak out his overflowing joy to everybody, and only wonders that all others should not feel just as he does. By and by he meets a repulse from an unexpected quarter. His feelings suddenly change; he distrusts his best convictions, and his despondency becomes as extreme as were his hope and joy.

In the high day of health and prosperity a Christian man of business gives his money and time and effort with cheerfulness and constancy for the cause of Christ. He has many friends; his look is full of sunshine; he infuses hope and life into everything he undertakes. By and by he loses health, loses property, loses his vivacity and hopefulness. Then his friends fall off; he slides out of his former social connections; he ceases to be recognized by some who once eagerly sought his friendship. Then he desponds, takes gloomy views of everything, judges others with severity, blames his best friends, is still more dissatisfied with himself, and

Bibliography

Butler, Jonathan. "The World of E. G. White and the End of the World." *Spectrum* (1979), 10(2):2–13.

Edersheim, Alfred. *Bible History: Old Testament.* Vols. 1–4. Grand Rapids, Mich.: Eerdmans, 1949 (reprint).

Fraser, G. E. *Diet, Life Expectancy, and Chronic Disease: Studies of Seventh-day Adventists and Other Vegetarians.* New York: Oxford University Press, 2003.

Fraser, G. E.; T. M. Strahan; J. Sabate; W. L. Beeson; and D. Kissinger. "Effects of Traditional Coronary Risk Factors on Rates of Incident Coronary Events in a Low Risk Population: the Adventist Health Study." *Circulation* (1992) 86:406–413.

Fraser, G. E., and D. J. Shavlik. "Ten Years of Life: Is It a Matter of Choice?" *Archives of Internal Medicine* (2001) 161:1645–1652.

Fredrickson, B. L. "The Value of Positive Emotions." *American Scientist* (2003) 91:330–335.

Hardinge, M. G. *A Physician Explains Ellen White's Counsel on Drugs, Herbs, and Natural Remedies.* Hagerstown, Md.: Review and Herald, 2001.

Kellogg, J. H. *The Home Hand-Book of Domestic Hygiene and Rational Medicine.* London: International Tract Society, 1899.

Key, T. J. A.; G. E. Fraser; M. Thorogood; P. Appleby; V. Beral; G. Reeves; M. L. Burr; J. Chang-Claude; R. Frentzel-Beyme; J. W. Kuzma; J. Mann; and K. McPherson. "Mortality in Vegetarians and Non-Vegetarians: Detailed Findings From a Collaborative Analysis of Five Prospective Studies." *American Journal of Clinical Nutrition* (1999) 70:516S–524S.

McAdams, D. R. "Ellen G. White and the Protestant Historians." Unpublished manuscript, Andrews University, 1974.

McAdams, D. R. "Shifting Views of Inspiration: Ellen G. White Studies in the 1970s." *Spectrum* (1980) 10(4):27–41.

McMahon, *D. Acquired or Inspired? Exploring the Origins of the Adventist Lifestyle* (Warburton, Australia: Signs Publishing Co., 2005). A CD in which McMahon describes his research accompanies the book.

McMillen, S. I. *None of These Diseases*. Grand Rapids, Mich.: Fleming H. Revell, 1984.

Mills, P. K.; W. L. Beeson; R. L. Phillips; and G. E. Fraser. "Cohort Study of Diet, Lifestyle, and Prostate Cancer in Adventist Men." *Cancer* (1989) 64:598–604.

Nichol, F. D. *Ellen G. White and Her Critics*. Hagerstown, Md.: Review and Herald, 1951.

Numbers, R. *Prophetess of Health: A Study of Ellen G. White*. New York: Harper and Row, Publishers, 1976.

Phillips, R. L.; J. W. Kuzma; W. L. Beeson; and T. Lotz. "Influence of Selection Versus Lifestyle on Risk of Fatal Cancer and Cardiovascular Disease Among Seventh-day Adventists." *American Journal of Epidemiology* (1980) 112:296–314.

Rea, W. T. *The White Lie*. Turlock, Calif.: M & R Publications, 1982.

Robertson, J. J. *The White Truth*. Nampa, Idaho: Pacific Press, 1981.

Snowdon, D. A.; R. L. Phillips; and G. E. Fraser. "Meat Consumption and Fatal Ischemic Heart Disease." *Preventive Medicine* (1984) 13:490–500.

Veltman, Fred. *Full Report on the Life of Christ Research Project*. <http://www.adventistarchives.org/doc_info.asp?DOC ID=1188.> (1988).

White, A. L. "Ellen G. White and Marriage Relations," Part 1. *The Ministry,* March 1969, 6–8, 26, 27.

White, A. L. "Ellen G. White and Marriage Relations," Part 2. *The Ministry,* April 1969, 19–21, 23.

White Estate. *A Critique of Prophetess of Health.* Silver Spring, Md.: The Ellen G. White Estate, 1976.

If you enjoyed this book, you'll enjoy these as well: